MW01503096

Dedicated to

Diana, Laurén, Michael and Bryan

(handwritten inscription)

LMB publications

www.themilforddentist.com

9-16-2010

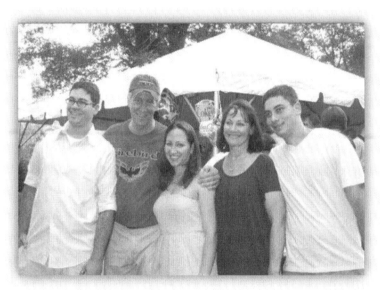

Michael, me, Laurén, Diana, Bryan

TABLE OF CONTENTS

Introduction

Surely you have heard a "good news /bad news" story. In my case, the good news is, I am still here and writing this next segment of *our* battle with cancer. The bad news is: *We* are still battling cancer. I use "we" deliberately because, even though I am the one with the physical illness, my family, friends and anyone connected with me is part of my army. They are my allies in this conflict, and **you** are now part of my private militia.

My first book, "Spiritual Signs and Lessons of a Survivor" concerned this life challenge with cancer and how spiritual signs helped guide me through the unimaginable tasks involved with it. Writing that manuscript was personally rewarding, enabling me to focus my thoughts and overcome my emotional and physical anguish. I wrote it for me, but as people began reading it they urged me to continue sharing the message and stories that gave them hope and encouragement in fighting their own issues.

The crux of my previous book revolved around spiritually gifted signs during and before cancer. In each story I address how help from a higher power aided with many of my life-changing decisions. We all have that connection, but we often do not look up and ask for guidance. Often we do not believe anyone is listening. Often we abandon the force that gladly helps. And, worst of all, we often will not look for, and therefore not see, the signs that can act as roadmaps directing us to safety.

My message is couched in real life stories. They should take you on an emotional rollercoaster, entertain you and drop you off at the end of each chapter with a few lessons I have learned concerning the events of that section of my life. They are my lessons that I have interpreted. I have been told by readers that they have their own view on my stories, and take away their own meanings. Please, be my guest, and imagine whatever lessons you believe fit with my narrative.

"The difference between school and life? In school, you're taught a lesson and then given a test. In life, you're given a test that teaches you a lesson." – Tom Bodett

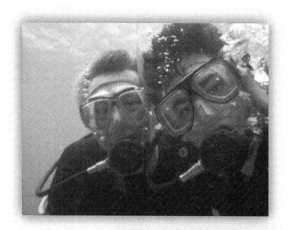

Me and Mike diving the Great Barrier Reef

Mike and me rafting the Tully River

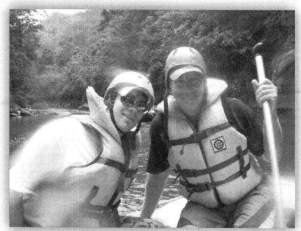

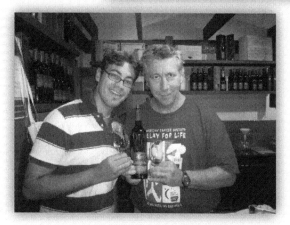

Mike and me wine tasting in the Barossa Valley

Australia: The Cancer Returns

This has to be the stupidest thing I have ever done, I thought as I crossed the Pacific Ocean heading to Australia: It may also be the last.

My stomach churned with mild discomfort, and the fact that I had not had a good bowel movement in two weeks played heavily on my mind – which was already dealing with the fact that **"the cancer"** had returned. Two years prior to this, I survived an eleven-hour surgery and 60 days of chemotherapy to treat a rare cancer of the appendix which had spread aberrant cells throughout my abdominal cavity. Unfortunately, some of these cells were now multiplying in several locations. The most damaging effect was the fact that one of these cancerous growths was strangling my colon. Whatever I ate was not fully passing through to the other end – the plumbing was backing up.

A week before boarding the plane, my oncologist sat with my wife, Diana, and me in an examination room. In her careful, delicate manner, Dr. Lacy informed us that my discomfort was caused by a recurrence of the disease, and indicated a need for surgery.

"How soon do we have to do this?" I asked.

"The sooner the better," she responded, stating the obvious.

"Can I die if I put off surgery for a month or so?"

"You should get the surgery as soon as you can, but it is probably not immediately life- threatening. You could have an episode where your colon would be totally blocked and that would necessitate immediate surgery," Dr. Lacy said. "Where are you planning on going?"

Dr. Lacy knew I was constantly on the go, and I would try to work my surgeries and treatments around my travel plans. My attitude had always been to enjoy every day and experience as much "life" as I could.

"My middle son, Michael, is finishing up his college semester abroad in Australia and I am going there for a few weeks touring, diving, whitewater rafting, traveling the Outback and we will be back in four weeks – at Christmas. I am supposed to leave in four days," I said.

Dr. Lacy looked at Diana, the most practical of our family, who implied with her look that going to the other side of the planet was not a good idea.

"I am not going with him," Diana said. "It is not my kind of adventure."

After more discussion concerning my options, Diana and I left.

Following some soul-searching and many tears, we agreed that even though going to Australia was not a good idea, it seemed like the right thing for me. Before making the final decision, we needed to consult with one of our dearest and smartest friends: It was time to call **The SMIK.** The SMIK is the nickname of Dr. Robert S. and it stands for The **S**martest **M**an **I** **K**now. Dr. Robert is not only an Massachusetts Institute of Technology graduate, a physician, an Eagle Scout, and an ideal father/husband, but his thought pattern combines reality, logic and knowledge wrapped in compassion and love.

" … Well that's the story," I said after downloading all of the new information concerning the cancer and my travel plans to The SMIK.

He was already up to date on my condition and had done considerable research on the disease and current treatments around the world. Dr. Robert had helped me through the first stage of the disease and was constantly involved with my progress.

"**Going** to Australia is probably not the smartest thing to do now, but if you are careful to eat moderately and maintain fluid intake, you should be able to return in one piece. I want you to enjoy your trip and do not worry about anything. However, as soon as you land back in the states, call me," he said, emphatically.

"*Not worrying about anything*" would be difficult, but knowing The SMIK would have some direction for me when I returned was a comfort to me and Diana.

The flight to Australia was long – very long. Fortunately, a sleeping pill enabled me to pass out for a good portion of the trip. However, during my waking moments, I managed to write a letter to Dr. Lacy and Dr. Salem (the doctor who performed my first eleven-hour surgery in July, 2005) concerning my disappointment in the medical profession after all these years of cancer research and modern technology. I felt there was absolutely no reason why my disease or any cancer could not be cured. Surgery, drugs and radiation seemed too limited in the scope of possible treatments. The medical profession needed some imagination. As a dentist, I have seen my profession nearly eliminate dental disease when certain standards of care are followed. In other cases, rehabilitation from dental disease is almost always possible, providing patients with health and function for the rest of their lives.

The following letter is unedited and slightly clouded by the sleeping pill, but I include it to show my actual state of being as I flew over the Pacific Ocean as well as when I completed it during my first day in Australia.

Dr. Lacy and Dr. Salem,

These are my thoughts as I fly to Australia having just found out that there seems to be a recurrent growth of suspicious cells within my abdominal cavity. Two years and two months ago, cellular material was removed from my innards, and a protocol was followed that seemed to be "the most up to date" and best tactic for the elimination of the current malady as well as the elimination of future problems. All parties involved understood that the Beast was a rare one and that unlike a dental cavity that has a definitive cause, treatment, and prognosis, this beast was more complicated.

Last time I allowed my creative process to take a back seat to what the medical community deemed reasonable and practical. I am in part a realist and know that medicine is advancing rapidly and our physicians have the best available technology and information and skill that can be expected. I further understand that advances in medicine do not always come from the established medical research community. One of the best innovations in my field of dentistry came from a dentist while he was caulking his windows in his home. He added some unique adaptations and transferred that caulking gun into what is today the state of the art technique for impression taking.

One definition of insanity is doing the same thing twice and expecting different results. I say this not as an affront to the path we are on, but as a challenge at this moment with this patient (me), to look a little outside of the box. You have read my book and I believe what I have written, and I have seen some signs that I cannot ignore. Certainly I do not understand them, but if I get them on paper, they may click with one of my caregivers and good things could happen.

(The entire body of this letter is omitted because of its length, but the ending portion accents the point of the letter which was completed after my first day in Australia.)

*I have the highest regard and inexhaustible faith and trust in Dr. Lacy and Dr. Salem, and know that they are using all of the appropriate avenues to keep me alive. It was not easy to sit here and write these straw grasping thoughts. But the reality is that I have pictured a path that we are going down, and it does not look like a yellow brick road. **Do I actually believe that we could come up with a creative innovative*** *cure for my malady? Do I actually believe that we could step out of the box and be successful with some crazy scheme? Do I sense every moment the urgency of my plight? Do I prey to God constantly? You know the answers.*

I have landed and went to the Australian zoo, and stayed for quite a while in the butterfly pavilion. As I looked at the few butterflies flapping about, I was obviously thinking about my plight. Analogies evolved simply as I watched these few flutterers. So few butterflies, so few cures for cancer..... Then a few more of the flying creatures appeared in my sight. They were there before, but I did not notice them. Yes they were camouflaged; and now a few more, and then some more. It seemed like I was uncovering hidden butterflies. But no, they were there, but I did not see what was right in front of me. Fifteen minutes later, the room was so full of these beauties that it seemed there was not a leaf without one. I moved to the indoor bird pavilion, and the same experience occurred. There are butterflies and birds and cures for cancer and they are staring us in the face. Please use the cures that we know of, and know that there are some butterflies, birds, or cures that are right in front of us waiting, fluttering, and chirping and at this moment in time begging to be noticed and used.

Thank you for your understanding, compassion and time.

Bob Rauch

The last paragraph in the letter is the most profound thought I have ever experienced. Standing in that pavilion and noticing butterflies multiplying exponentially simply by **really** opening my eyes, empowered me more than any other life experience I have ever had. The next two weeks with Michael were full of butterflies, birds and belief that I would be cured.

I met Michael the next day in Sydney Australia, and we began our journey. The itinerary was jam-packed with physical, mental and spiritual challenges and revelations.

I did not tell Michael the cancer had returned until we landed back in New York. He took the news well, but did not seem to believe this would be a terminal problem. He had faith that I would jump this hurdle as I had jumped all of the previous hurdles that confronted me. I called Diana and she was overjoyed that we were back on this continent and urged me to get off the phone and call The SMIK immediately. I did.

"Bob, welcome home," he said. "I have made calls all around the country and have found the two doctors that I want you to see. I have made appointments for you: One next week at Sloan-Kettering hospital; and the other appointment with Dr. Sugarbaker in Washington, D.C., the following Friday."

"Thank you so much," I responded with relief, knowing Dr. Robert had done hours of research and had jump-started my motion. It was not a clear cut path, but it was a direction.

Lessons:

Ask for help from those you trust and know more than you do. Advice from friends and relatives may sometimes be worthwhile, but advice from a SMIK is priceless.

Having cancer **does not** mean: Stop everything and prepare to die. It means: Go on with life as you have planned. While you are doing that, investigate solutions and prepare to march forward with the strength and resolution that you will overcome your illness. The batter is not out until the last strike is in the catcher's glove.

When the final strike is pitched and you are certain that the end of your time at the plate is at hand, you are not giving up. You are walking off the field with dignity and looking forward to the next game at a different ball field.

Cancer can be defeated. Every day new modalities are found. As we open our field of vision we will see more butterflies, birds and cures for cancer.

"The journey of a thousand miles begins with the first step." – Chinese proverb.

Visit Australia.

The Direction

The consultation with the doctors at Memorial Sloan-Kettering Cancer Center was unrewarding at best. They suggested the same surgical procedure I had done two years before: open my abdomen, wash it with saline (water) solution, followed by intravenous chemotherapy for six months. That procedure had already been done by one of the finest surgeons in the country, and it did not eliminate all of the cancer. We left there and called The SMIK.

"Well Bob, that seems to be the standard technique for your disease. But Dr. Sugarbaker, who you will be seeing next week, has a few twists that he adds to the procedure. Call me on your way home from your consultation in Washington, D.C. next week, and we will review our options. Remember, we are in *gathering information* mode now; we will make decisions and choose a definitive direction after we get as much data as we can," the SMIK said as we ended our conversation.

Diana and I anxiously looked forward to our consultation with Dr. Sugarbaker for several reasons: We wanted an alternative treatment to the Sloan-Kettering suggestion; and we wanted a weekend away together. The consultation would be sandwiched between a visit to our son Michael at Goucher College in Townsend, Maryland and a visit to our daughter, Laurén at Georgetown Law in D.C..

Time marches on and – in our case – it seemed to be going at warp speed. Before we knew it, our weekend getaway was over and we were done with Dr. Sugarbaker's consultation.

As promised, we called The SMIK.

"What did Dr. Sugarbaker have to say?" he asked.

I talked for over an hour, explaining all about the consultation while Diana drove. I informed him of Dr. Sugarbaker's wife, and office manager, Ilse, and how kind and helpful she was. She was also very impressed with The SMIK's persistence and determination in getting an appointment for me.

The SMIK appreciated the pleasantries, but moved the conversation along and solicited solid information concerning treatment and prognosis from Dr. Sugarbaker's viewpoint.

"His treatment is similar to the other hospitals in the fact that he would open me up, remove any cancerous tissue and after about eleven hours of surgery he would put me back together and sew me up," I said. The main difference between him and the other surgeons is that while he had me open, he would be washing my organs and insides with heated chemicals that would come in direct contact with any microscopic cancer cells that were left behind. He seemed like a very conscientious and intelligent man."

"He is one of the most, if not the most, published and respected specialists concerning this particular type of cancer." The SMIK informed me. "Not only has he written most of the relevant information about this disease, but he has probably done more operations of this kind than anyone on the planet. I am familiar with the heated chemotherapy during his surgery, and there is some dispute as to whether or not it is effective. Insurance companies think that it is experimental and will probably not pay for that part of the procedure. But whether or not they pay is not important right now. From a logical medical viewpoint, the technique makes perfect sense."

The SMIK then coaxed me to relate almost every detail about our meeting again. He asked Diana how she felt about our meeting. He asked us more questions that seemed to draw out more information. Then, like a seasoned lawyer, he asked:

"Do you think that surgery is the correct course of action?"

"Yes," Diana and I answered.

"Do you think that the procedure at Yale or Sloan Kettering can cure you?"

"No," we answered.

"Do you think that Dr. Sugarbaker can cure you?"

"Yes," we responded.

We started the process over again from the beginning and ended with the same directional questions. By the time we reached New Jersey, halfway home, we had made a decision and were ready to move forward.

The process of arriving at our decision was much easier than it had appeared when we left Washington, D. C. The clarity and correctness of our choice was so evident to us that it did not need to be overanalyzed. It was the correct decision given the information available to us at the time, and we felt comfortable with it.

Fortunately, Dr. Sugarbaker had a cancellation in his busy schedule, and had one opening for a surgery six weeks from the day of our initial consultation. After that, he was booked for another six weeks: too long to wait.

That one-day opening in his schedule was a gift to me from above. Now all we had to do was make sure I survived another six weeks until the surgery, and pray that this time all of the cancer cells would be eliminated.

Lessons:

The greatest source of direction comes from gathering as much information as you can on the subject. You can then thoroughly and systematically map out plans to explore. Each path will have benefits, risks and probably some unknown consequences. The more you rethink and add solid information into the equations, the clearer your decision will be. Rarely will one path be the perfect road; but after considerable analysis, one path will be better. Choose it and move forward. You can usually change your course if new information presents itself, but hopefully you have done your homework well enough before you started choosing your direction. A sailboat without direction will flounder in the wind and end up on the rocks. Stay off the rocks.

There is always a chance that there may be an opening for you to be seen by someone who is "totally booked."

You are allowed to be seen by "the best." Pleasant persistence promotes possibilities, especially if they are punctuated with prayer.

There is no better gift that can be had in a lifetime than friendship. We love our Dr. Robert, and the fact that he is the SMIK is just whipped cream on the strawberry shortcake of life's gift to us.

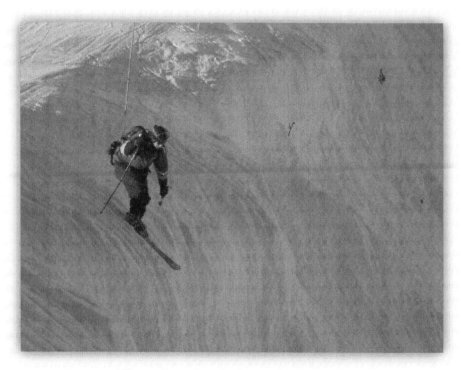

"Some bonehead always jumps in."

The Flight Attendant Angel

For the past twenty years, my neighbor Billy and I have gone out west for a week-long ski trip. Jackson Hole, Wyoming, Vail, Colorado, Park City, Utah, and Whistler, British Columbia, are just a few of our favorite spots. The list is impressive and the stories priceless. As the years went on, other friends joined, and our troop usually consisted of six to eight on our yearly jaunt.

One year in Jackson Hole, we all lined our ski tips along a cliff, peering at the steep incline below. Without a word, Billy jumped off the cliff edge and proceeded down the slope, vanishing into the trees below.

"Some bonehead always jumps in," said Timothy. The next moment, Timothy jumped off, leaving three of us staring at a nearly sixty degree leap into a sea of fresh powder followed by a wall of trees and the unknown. Naturally we all followed suit, one bonehead after another.

We have been the *Boneheads* ever since. (Look for our matching hats, jerseys, and shirts on the hill the next time you go skiing.)

Billy Ho, another of our group, would research where we should go and set us up with luxury accommodations: including chefs, chauffeurs, mountainside mansions and plenty of extras. The Bonehead ski week was an annual trip I looked forward to all year. I had never missed one, even the year after my first cancer surgery in 2005. That year, we skied in Vermont because the Boneheads knew an "out west" trip would have been too much for this Bonehead to handle. Even though I only skied one day in Killington, my perfect record was in tact.

With my new diagnosis of cancer in November, and our scheduled surgery with Dr. Sugarbaker set for February 12, I would still be able to go on this year's Bonehead trip set for the last week in January. Overriding Diana's objections, I packed my bags.

The limousine picked Billy, Timothy, Ed, Don, Dave and me up at my house at four o'clock in the morning on January 26 beginning our trip to Lake Tahoe in Nevada. This legendary ski destination has some of the steepest and most rugged terrain in the country, and is famous for the abundance of fresh powder that comes during the frequent "dumping" of snow. It was also the first place Billy and I went when we started our trips out west 20 years before.

All of the guys had been warned by their wives, as well as Diana, to look out for me and make sure that I did not endanger myself on any ski hills. Every Bonehead knew my cancer had returned and I was fragile. This trip was beyond the scope of what was reasonable and rational for a man whose abdomen was ready to explode. They all agreed to keep a close eye on me, knowing I would not be dissuaded from going skiing with the Boneheads.

Once again, my colon was getting blocked up, and as long as I limited my food intake, I figured that the discomfort and distention of my gut would not be a major issue during the Bonehead trip.

I was wrong.

As usual, the trip was a blast. We laughed, *they* ate and we skied almost every day in fresh powder, sometimes as deep as three feet. Memorable runs like the Wall at Kirkwood Mountain Resort, the Face and Mott Canyon at Heavenly, combined with evenings at the casino in the town of Lake Tahoe only added to the great time with great friends.

By the end of the week, however, my medical condition had taken a turn for the worse. Even though I tried to hide my discomfort from my friends, everyone was aware that on the last day I was having intense pain. I would have given away my last dime if only I could empty my colon. The plumbing had totally backed up and any food I had eaten during my week away (which was mostly baby food and soup) had not exited. By now, my abdomen was distended and even sitting down required jockeying into a certain position to avoid deep-seated excruciating pain.

The first leg of the trip home was from the Reno, Nevada, airport to Denver, Colorado. The short flight was an exercise in agony. My six-foot two-inch frame has trouble sitting in airplane seats on my best day. In my compromised state, sitting in row *twenty* without any free space to move brought me almost to tears. Getting off the plane in Denver, my emotions switched from relief to fear for the next leg of the journey. Fortunately, the plane was delayed for several hours and I was able to lie down on the airport terminal floor to regroup. Ed brought me some water and offered me something to eat, and fashioned a bed for me out of Bonehead jackets. The other Boneheads hovered around and tried to comfort me, but there was little they could do. We finally boarded the plane for the four hour flight from Denver to New York, and as fate would have it, we proceeded to wait on the tarmac for another forty-five minutes. By the time we readied for take-off, I had reached the end of my ability to hold it together.

During our time waiting for takeoff, the Boneheads befriended the flight attendant, as we normally do. Our bright-red Bonehead shirts combined with our entertaining antics made us more than just passengers. One of the flight attendants noticed my anguish and asked if there was anything she could do to make me more comfortable. I am sure my wincing face and contorted body communicated the situation better than the words.

"Is there any way I could lay down in the galley area where you get the food from, near the front of the plane?" I asked, not expecting her to comply with such a ridiculous request. I furthered my case by explaining briefly about my cancer, the upcoming surgery and the problem I was presently experiencing.

"We will be taking off in a few minutes, but after we are in the air I will see what I can do," she said with compassion and hope in her voice.

It seemed like hours of throbbing abdominal cramping had passed when she returned. It was actually less than ten minutes after takeoff.

"Follow me," she said, directing me to the front of the plane past the curtain separating our section from the first class passengers, then to the galley situated just behind the cockpit. She lay down some blankets and at least half a dozen pillows. With no more urging, I curled up on the floor and settled into my in-flight bed. The flight attendants worked around me and constantly checked on my condition. The one who brought me there heated a water bottle and gave it to me to place on my stomach. The warmth somewhat eased my pain and she replaced the bottle several times throughout the flight. Her compassion and concern for my well-being was over the top. She cared for me with the warmth and tenderness of a mother to a sick child.

"I am so sorry," she said as the pilot announced that we were preparing to land. "You have to return to your seat for landing."

The four-hour flight was far from comfortable, but with the help of this saintly woman I had made it through.

"You cannot imagine what you have done for me," I said with tears welling at the corners of my eyes.

"You cannot imagine what you have given me," She replied, tears rolling down her cheeks.

Obviously, I was confused. She had allowed me to break, I am sure many rules about letting passengers sleep in the galley, had fashioned a bed for me, provided hot water bottles and even had the pilots and other flight attendants treat me like royalty. Now, she was thanking me?

"Why are you thanking me?" I asked

"Well," she began, "A year ago, my mother died of cancer. I was very busy flying around the country and managing my family. I never imagined that she was really dying and did not spend the time with her that I should have. I have been feeling guilty about that since her death. I miss my mom and think about her all the time. When I saw you sitting in the seat and in pain, and learned that you were suffering from cancer, a vision of my mom crossed my mind. While I took care of you for the past four hours, I pictured that I was really taking care of my mom. You gave me the chance to care for her, through you. Does that make any sense?"

"Absolutely," I said, as I put my arms around her and we shared a long, rewarding hug.

Lessons:

There are nice people in the world that will go out of their way to help someone in need. Imagine if everyone had as much compassion for a stranger as that flight attendant had for me.

Be sure you have a few Boneheads in your life. Friends are the spices and seasonings of life's buffet.

You do not have to have a perfect record of "annual trips never missed." Sometimes it is okay to stay home. In hindsight, I was a real Bonehead to have gone on that trip.

Food for a Dying Man

For one week after returning from the Bonehead ski trip, I tried to overcome my discomfort while ignoring what was turning into a real life crisis. Even though I was confident that the upcoming surgery would alleviate my pain as well as eliminate the cancerous growths, each day was becoming harder and harder to get along. I was becoming weaker (obviously from lack of nutritional intake), and on that Friday (six days after my trip), I went with Diana to see Dr. Lacy concerning my immediate abdominal pain. She called the surgeon, Dr. Sugarbaker, and they agreed I should be checked into the hospital immediately in order to get some nutrition. My body was shutting down and would not be in any shape for the surgery if it did not get fed.

By Friday at five o'clock in the afternoon, I was in a room at Yale-New Haven Hospital and looking forward to being fed intravenously. Inserting a "PICC line" is a relatively common procedure. It seems like a logical way to get food into the bloodstream if your mouth/stomach/colon rout is not working. A tube is placed into a vein on the inside of your arm and is connected to liquid food from a large plastic bag, and your body receives balanced nutrition without the need to pass from the mouth to the other end.

After insufficient nourishment for several weeks, I was looking forward to getting something to eat even though I would not taste or smell it. I had not eaten anything at all for two days, and only had soup, Jell-O or baby food for the past three weeks. Every minute seemed like eternity while waiting for the PICC line to be placed. I was literally starving.

"What do you mean I can't get a PICC line tonight?" I asked the nurse, rather perturbed.

"Well," she said, "there is a special team that places the PICC line into patients and they only work in the hospital until five on weekdays, and it is now five-thirty. They will be back on Monday."

"Are you kidding me?" I snapped.

"I am sorry sir," she continued, "but that is the way the PICC line is administered. However, in the event of an emergency, there is a team in the Interventional Radiology department that can also place the PICC line."

"This is an emergency!" I quickly responded, "I cannot stay in this hospital until Monday morning when the PICC line team returns. That is two more days without food!"

"Well, if your doctor informs us that it is an emergency, we will try to work you into the schedule with the IR department," she replied.

"How late are they here?" I asked feeling a sense of urgency getting to them before **they** went home too.

"Oh, they are there all night for trauma patients and emergency procedures," the nurse responded.

That was the first bit of good news I had all day. I would call Dr. Lacy and have her connect with the nurse, and I would have my PICC line and food in an hour or two: Dinner by eight. Dr. Lacy was not easily reached, but within an hour we had the necessary paperwork to get me the PICC line on an emergency basis. I waited for another two hours before bothering my nurse again and asked why I did not have my procedure yet. She told me they are usually busy in that department and as soon as they had a few free moments for this minor procedure – which would take less than thirty minutes – they would send for me.

"It shouldn't be too long," she said with a smile.

By eleven that night, I confronted my nurse again and told her I was going to bed and I looked forward to being awakened at any hour of the night to get my PICC line. I then put a large note on my door: **"Waiting for my PICC line, please wake me up."** I shut my eyes and went to bed starving, but hopeful that within the next few hours I would be wheeled downstairs and have nutrients cruising through my body by morning. Surely the IR department would have some time during the night to see this starving man.

There is a difference between the luxury of hunger and the illness of starvation. At this point, I was making the transition between the two. Sure I was hungry, but my body was now in cannibal mode and the stored food within my cellular tissue was being actively utilized. They say a person can go up to six weeks without food, but the process causes changes in your body and mind before the real dangers of body shut down occur.

The first change for me came in my attitude and my inability to control my frustration. I woke up Saturday morning paged my nurse and, with considerable bitterness, began to interrogate her.

"Why didn't I get a PICC line yet? I've been here for eight hours!" I demanded.

It was now seven in the morning and it seemed impossible that the IR department had not had a break all night for my simple procedure.

"You need to get them to get me down to IR right now!" I continued.

This was not my normal tact for getting things done. I have always used the kind; *you get more bees with honey* approach. This was the angry, irate, *pain-in-the-butt patient* approach that rarely works, but my self control was no longer in place.

"They are aware that you need a PICC line and I am sure that you are on the list to get one today," she said without conviction.

She was useless. I needed to go to the next level. I asked to see the doctor on the floor and got nowhere with him, either. Then I called Dr. Lacy, and hit another dead end with her being unable to expedite the procedure. By eleven that morning, I felt abandoned. I was just another body in a bed, and would be treated when my paperwork caught the eye of someone in the IR department. My pain and plight was real to no one but me.

The countless times I have seen emergency patients in pain in my dental practice by fitting them into the schedule or coming in on evenings and weekends should count for *something* in the cosmic world, I thought. I wanted to call in the celestial return for the good deeds I had done.

Just then, I started to laugh out loud. The solution came to me like a flash of light in the middle of a dark night. I asked for help from above and He gave me the open door I would now pass through. I picked up my cell phone and dialed the hospital's main number.

"Hello, this is Yale University Hospital, how may I direct your call?" answered a voice at the other end.

"This is Dr. Rauch," I said, "And I would like to be connected with the head of the IR department."

I would routinely use my "Doctor" title for dinner reservations, but this time I knew I had stretched the use of my dental degree beyond its intended limit.

"Hello, IR department," the voice said, cold and distant.

"May I speak with the department head please?" I asked.

"This is he."

"What is your name?" I asked.

My dad had taught me to always communicate with the person in charge and to be sure to get his or her name. If you need to avoid protocol policy, this is a good start. Policies are needed and usually should be followed, but there are definitely times when policy should be bypassed. I believed this was one of them.

"Dr. B., and who is this?" he responded with a hint of annoyance in his tone.

"This is Dr. Rauch, and I have a patient in room 506 who needs a PICC line, stat."

I love the word stat. It is one of those doctor code words that mean "immediately." I was sure the word would convey that I was a medical caregiver, as well as accenting the urgency of a PICC line for the patient in room 506.

"A PICC line stat?" he barked. "Why?"

"The patient is having a major operation in two weeks and has not eaten adequately for the past three weeks. He is starving and bodily functions are starting to shut down," I said. *That will convince him of the reason for a "stat PICC line,"* I thought.

"Who is this?" he asked again.

"Dr. Rauch," I said confidently.

"What is the patient's name?" he asked with some frustration.

I hesitated for a moment then answered tangentially.

"He is in room 506."

"What is his name?" he asked again sternly.

"Bob Rauch."

The ten second silence was deafening.

"Are you the patient?" he asked, direct and forcefully.

"Yes," I said sheepishly.

"This is unacceptable! Patients do not call up heads of departments requesting services. You have your doctor go through proper channels –"

I cut him off. "I haven't eaten in over three weeks!" I began, then pleaded my case.

"This is not how it is done," he said before curtly ending our conversation.

Not good. **Not good at all**, I thought, contemplating what the consequences of my actions could be. Then I resigned myself to put my medical scheduling in the hands of God. I should have done that sooner. Twenty minutes after my conversation with Dr. B., a nurse came into the room with a portable bed, and took me to the IR department for my PICC line.

Now I was a little worried that I had pissed off the guy who was going to do the surgery on me. That could be even worse than upsetting the waiter in a restaurant before he brings you your food. Nah, I thought, doctors are professionals and would not be emotionally driven or easily upset by bad patient behavior … or would they? I was greeted in the IR surgery room mildly by Dr. B. and warmly by his assisting nurse.

"Hello, Dr. Rauch," she said enthusiastically. I had seen her several times a few years prior, when I was having my first cancer adventures. "Did you finish that book you were working on?" she asked with much interest.

"Yes! And I have a copy waiting for you after I get my PICC line placed," I said relieved, knowing Dr. B. had overheard our conversation. Her acknowledgement of me as a doctor and someone special who she remembered gave me some credence as being someone who was not just an annoying, over-reactive patient. As soon as I returned to my room after the procedure and had food flowing into my veins, I signed and sent a copy of my first book to the nurse and Dr. B.

Lessons:

Policies and protocol are in place to make an organization more efficient and more capable of providing the services they render. If at all possible, follow their rules and systems. Working within the confines of the establishment will often get you to where you need to go.

Sometimes you have to take charge. ***The squeaky wheel gets the oil.*** It is not wrong to ask for what you need regarding medical care. The worst that can happen is you get yelled at. The best is that you might get what you need.

Be nice to nurses (and all caregivers). You will probably see them again, and if they remember you with a smile, that's a good thing.

If you are having discomfort or any medical issue, do not wait until the symptoms have reached beyond your pain threshold to seek professional help. Routine procedures can quickly turn into emergencies.

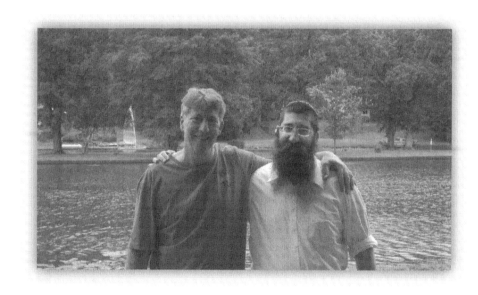

Me & Sion

The Surgery

This was my second surgery of this type, which involved cutting me open from just below my rib cage to just below my belly button. The twelve-inch-long incision would reveal most of my organs including: stomach, liver, small and large intestine and everything else located in my midsection. Dr. Sugarbaker would manipulate the body parts in such a way as to cleanse any cancerous cells that were present with a knife, chemicals, and scrub brush. His job would take him and his team around eleven hours. He is a meticulous artist who gives superhuman attention to his mission. However, as fine a surgeon as he is, my healing and survival would rely on "higher powers."

The morning of the surgery found Diana, Laurén, Michael and me quietly preparing for my procedure. Mike was down from college in Baltimore and Laurén was in her first year of law school only twenty minutes down the road in D.C. Soon, I would kiss them goodbye and be rolled into the operating room. We said very little, but held hands, shared hugs and held back our tears to show each other our strength and faith all would go well. Obviously there was a chance I would never get off the operating table, or that all of the cancer could not be removed, or hundreds of other complications could occur. We did not need to discuss the "what if" scenarios. Plans were in place in the event of problems, but for now all thoughts were directed to success.

I had the easy job. Once the sedative took effect, all I needed to do was wake up after the last stitch was in place. Dr. Sugarbaker's job was difficult, but he had done this hundreds of times before, and this is what he did best. My family and friends had the toughest job. I had sent out an e-mail to all of my contacts asking them to pray for me at selected times throughout the day. There is no medical evidence those prayers helped my recovery, but trust me, they did.

My family was seated in the waiting room for eleven hours dealing with fears of my mortality at the edge of their emotional stability. The fact that they had each other, and knowing that people all over the planet were praying for me, offered them some solace. However, they still were waiting anxiously for news of my progress the entire day. Mike had to return to Baltimore but remained in touch with his mom and sister for any news.

When Dr. Sugarbaker finally came out of the operation and entered their room, Diana and Laurén breathed a full breath, leaned forward and waited for his words as well as the tone of his voice.

"He is recovering and the procedure went well," Dr. Sugarbaker said. "He is still sedated, but you can go in and wait with him while he wakes up. The results of the surgery – whether or not we removed all of the cancer – will be determined after the pathologist gives his report in a day or two. Until then, I feel confident that your husband tolerated the operation well and that I removed all of the cancer."

Even though Dr. Sugarbaker was tired from his eleven hours of work and unemotional with the data he shared, he made my girls feel comfortable in the fact that I would be a "survivor."

I was still oblivious to everything. I had a tube in my mouth forcing me to breath; intravenous tubes in both of my forearms pumping drugs and other life fluids into my veins; three drainage tubes in my abdomen which looked like rubber test tubes protruding from my belly; a catheter in my private part so I did not wet myself; a tube in my nose extending to my stomach that prevented any fluids form entering my colon, which would not be working for about a week; fifty stitches extending from my chest to my pubis; duct tape-like material wrapped around me holding everything in place; and to top it off, my belly button had been removed. That's right, I have no belly button.

Diana and the kids were drained physically and emotionally by this time, but they needed to get me through the next few hours. I would wake up in unbelievable agony (even with the pain meds maxed out) strapped to a recovery bed and totally disoriented. This would be a tough task for them to handle.

"Danny … Terry …" Diana stammered. She recognized the couple that crossed her path as she headed to the recovery room.

Danny and Terry have been our friends for over 30 years. They have not lived near us for at least 15 years, but we still communicate with them several times a year. They lived in Maryland, about half an hour from Washington Hospital Center and my e-mail gave them a sign that they should not just pray for me, but should show up at the hospital and be there if they were needed. They are incredibly strong, spiritually-oriented people who we love dearly. We never requested anyone to be there during the operation, but their presence was a gift from above to

Diana and the kids. Unbeknownst to us, they had also added me to their church prayer list, forwarded my e-mail to their global network and had "Pray for Bob Rauch" bracelets made up that were being worn by hundreds in their community.

"How did it go?" Danny asked, with the compassion of a minister.

"We are going to see him now. Would you come with us?" Diana responded, knowing she could use some fresh emotional support at this time. Their answer was obvious as they hugged her and proceeded into the recovery room.

I must have looked pretty scary with tubes, tape and a colorless ashen face that was contorted with suffering. Diana had trouble looking at me, so Terry consoled her while Danny remained with Laurén, gently holding my hand, consciously avoiding the surrounding tubes and wires.

"Make sure that he does not rip out the breathing tube. It is very painful, but he will need to keep it in place for at least another half hour," the nurse told those surrounding me. I don't think I could have removed it anyway, because my arms were strapped down to the side rails.

I am not sure just how much pain I was in, but fortunately most of that block of time is deleted form my active memory banks. I do remember, however, the first moment of true consciousness.

"Do you want to play some golf?" Danny asked me earnestly.

His dry sense of humor was not wasted on the near-dead. I am sure I answered in the affirmative and promised to give him a golf thrashing that he would never forget. What I actually said was so incoherent he just smiled and lovingly continued clutching my hand. The tube down my throat burned like a thousand torches and prevented any comprehensible speech.

The next two days were a blur for me, but Diana was the glue that kept things from tearing at the seams. She watched over me and left my side only when Laurén could stand the post. Laurén went back and forth to the hospital daily, taking care of both her father and her mother while doing her best to stay on top of her schoolwork. Michel was back at college and would come down on the weekends, while Bryan was in Connecticut managing our home and taking care of Nana and the dog. The nurses were all excellent and the fact that Diana filled them with Godiva chocolates, gourmet cookies flowers, and food only added to their appreciation of me as a patient.

There are moments during the cloudy times of recovery that the patient has indescribable thoughts. They rush between appreciation for family friends and life, and cross to the other side of emotion and enter the dark zone: Why do I have to suffer with this pain and what does my future hold? Those questioning times are when we are more receptive to forces other than what we see, hear, smell, taste or touch. For me, it was time to talk with God and listen to His answers.

The belief in the existence of a supreme power has been a source of anxiety, confusion, and doubt and has often created problems between people since the dawn of time. Fortunately, many people are secure in their faith and believe God exists. Some people are still searching. Thankfully for me, I have no doubts. My concept of God may not be exactly the same as anyone else's, but I take comfort in the fact that He exists and that He is my friend. As my friend, He knows what my needs are and if I ask Him for assistance, He will provide it for me – usually in an unexpected way. He is obviously very creative, and even though He has the ability to just handle the problems, He has chosen to share insights and let me figure out my own solutions.

About four or five days into my recovery, I was alone and began a conversation with my friend, God. I could no longer hold back the tears of pain, grief and worry. I did not want my family to be crushed by the weight of me crumbling in front of them the next morning. Exhaustion had overtaken me, and I could not see withstanding another hour of what my senses were confronting. I needed God to show Himself in more than a far-reaching interpretation of something that may be a sign of His presence. Like a crying child, I needed Him to physically hug me and hold my hand. My faith was the last thing holding me together, and that was waning fast.

An obvious question you might have here would be: "If God were your friend and could do anything, why would He give you cancer in the first place? Why would He make His friend suffer and why doesn't He just cure you?"

The answer that works for me is probably best described using a rather nontheistic analogy. My friend, Ed, is a much better golfer than I am, but I would not ask him to hit my golf ball and count it as my score. My friend, Billy, is a much better skier than I am, but I would not have him ski the mountain for me. My friend, God, can create anything and do anything in life for me, but I would not want Him to live my life for me. I do however; ask Ed's advice in golf, Billy's advice in skiing and God's advice in life.

The analogy might be viewed as weak when overanalyzed, but when you factor in the issue of free will, this viewpoint works for me. I must include here the fact that, even though I felt comfortable with my relationship and friendship with God, there is no doubt that He is God. He is "THE MAN": all powerful, all knowing and I respect and love Him so very much.

As if on cue from the director of a play, a nurse came in just after I finished my monologue with God asking Him for a physical sign showing me that He was still by my side. I had lain the gauntlet down, and it was His turn to respond. Like leaving a message on a friend's answering machine, it was His turn to pick up the phone and give me a call.

"It's time for your Heparin shot," the nurse said lifting my shirt and puncturing my abdomen, injecting the fluid that stopped blood clots from forming. Then she adjusted my nose/stomach tube, and took my blood pressure and temperature. If that was God's return call, I was not impressed. A little more pain had just been added to my already fragile state. Fortunately, the nurse also gave me more pain medication and sleeping pills that got me through the rest of the night.

The answer to my Godly request met me in the hallway the next day. Sion, the man in a room across the hall from me, was recovering from the same surgery as me. He was at least ten years younger than me, and was operated on a week before mine. He had already taken walks in the halls and said "hello" to me as I exited my room for the first time. We both had tubes and wires hanging from metal rolling poles. Leaning on our poles enabled us to take one agonizing step at a time.

He is a Hasidic Jew who follows the biblical teachings as they were taught in ancient times. His dress, speech and views are distinctive, and this would usually not promote easy interaction with someone who was not also Hasidic, especially a Jewish man who had married out of the faith. We crossed paths again later that day and shared our commonalities. We had the same surgeon, the same disease, similar roots (Brooklyn, N. Y.) and shared some basics of our religion. That was the total of what we had in common on the surface.

Though his Hebrew accent was thick, I was able to understand that he wanted to perform a religious ceremony with me that evening before sunset. The ceremony is called Tefillin and I vaguely remembered what it was about from my childhood. After my Bar Mitzvah at age thirteen, I minimized my connections with formal religion. Being a product of the 1960's, and assimilating into the eclectic religious times, Tefillin was dropped as part of any routine. The ten- minute procedure is supposed to be performed in the morning and symbolizes one's connectedness to God. You bind your heart and hands to His service and on a daily basis affirm that He will always be part of your life.

Ask and you shall receive. It did not take much imagination for me to believe this was my return call from above. Obviously, I accepted his offer.

Sion explained the procedure as he wrapped the long leather ribbons around my fragile body, and we said the customary prayers that I vaguely recalled from childhood. I felt fulfilled and thanked him for sharing his prayer time with me.

"No, Robert, thank you," Sion said. "You see, by you allowing me to do something to help you, it fulfills my need to help others."

The logic was a little dizzying in my state but is crystal clear on the macro level of what God would wants each of us to do for others: offer the spiritual and personal hug in a time if extreme need. That evening I slept well, knowing God was bound firmly to my hand and heart and my request for a hug had been magnificently answered.

Two years later, Sion confided in me that just before his operation, he read a passage in the Bible that directed him to look for someone in need of his assistance. I guess that must have been me.

Lessons:

Before surgery, get your affairs in order. Communicate with your insurance broker (life, health, disability), accountant, banker (investment advisor), lawyer (estate planner), office manager (*Paulette*), all of your affiliated doctors and as many friends as you feel need and should know what is going on in your life.

Some old customs, like Tefillin, can be incredibly useful and put life into perspective: I guess that is why they are still around.

Sion and I talk often, and on Sukos (a Jewish holiday celebrating unity between people), I visit him and his family in Brooklyn. We eat, laugh and dance in the streets with more than a thousand other celebrants.

There is always room for new friends, even if your living styles are worlds apart.

Our healing process is aided greatly by the support of our friends and family. Their positive energy has power that is immeasurable. Danny and Terry are only two of the hundreds that aided in my healing process. Emails and phone messages reminded me daily of the love and support of my friends.

In the darkest night or when you are standing alone on the verge of desperation, you will always have a friend by your side. Just say hello and He will answer. That's what friends do.

Cyberknife

One year after my second eleven-hour surgery and twelve more rounds of chemotherapy, Dr. Lacy once again had bad news to share with Diana and me. The blood tests I was getting on a monthly basis showed increasing levels of a protein indicating the cancer cells were still present and growing. These protein levels, known as "tumor markers" are not always accurate, but when combined with my last abdominal CT scan, there was no escaping the gravity of the moment: I still had cancer.

"What are my options?" I asked in a cold, calculated, unemotional tone. I was suppressing my tears for my own sanity, as well as trying to keep Diana from breaking down and feeling hopeless.

"We could try some more chemotherapy," Dr. Lacy replied, unconvincingly. "We could consider going in again surgically. But the location of the cancer is precarious, and would be difficult for the surgeon to assault. It is in between the lobes of the liver and resting very close to a major artery and vein. I am looking into some other techniques that might work in this particular case."

"Like what?" I asked

"Well there is Radio Frequency Ablation, CyberKnife, and Gamma Knife. I am meeting with our cancer board next week to discuss your case in detail and will let you know what we think is the best option after our meeting," she said with some enthusiasm, but little certainty if any of the mentioned treatments would work.

Once again, Diana and I were leaving the doctor's office as if we had just gone 12 rounds with Muhammad Ali: banged up and thoroughly beaten. We went back home to lick our wounds and try to regain our faith and strength. Tomorrow we would make some calls and enlist our troops for the forthcoming battle. That night we made no calls and let the phone ring without answering it. We hugged, cried and hugged some more. Few words were spoken; none were needed.

The first call at eight o'clock the next morning was to The SMIK.

"Get a pen and paper," the SMIK said after I told him my current status and what Dr. Lacy had discussed at our meeting the previous day.

"Put the letters A, B and C on the pages and leave some room under each heading."

Aristotle would be proud of the SMIK. Dr. Robert S. used logic like a precision instrument. He would lay out the options: surgery, chemotherapy, radiation, or nothing. Then, he described the risks and rewards of each. We discussed and re-discussed the options, adding and subtracting benefits and drawbacks on each re-clarification. By the end of the hour-long conversation, I had a paper with a list of tasks to perform and a direction with hope and possibilities at its end.

"Bob, What you are going through now is **not** immediately life-threatening, and I believe that we will get through this episode and you will continue to survive," the SMIK said near the end of our conversation. We talked for a little longer until he was sure my spirits were fired up and ready for the road ahead.

"What I need to do now," he continued, "is to talk to Diana."

Just when I was sure the SMIK was The Smartest Man I Know, he got even smarter. He knew Diana's heart was beaten up. She needed to hear there was hope and that I would be around for many years to come. He talked to her for another hour and I saw her face lighten up as he poured his loving essence into her over the phone line.

When they were done talking, Diana and I hugged and held each other for some time before I took my paper and proceeded to handle the tasks on my list.

The first call was to Dr. Sugarbaker. The comforting voice of his wife/secretary, Ilse, said he had already seen the reports and the CT scan from Dr. Lacy. Dr. Sugarbaker confirmed what I already knew; an operation in the particular area of my liver was not a good option. The cancer cells were located in an area inaccessible to his blade. Furthermore, he did not believe chemotherapy would be of any value either.

"This particular cancer does not usually invade into the tissue that it is connected to. It is possible that you can live a long life without these cells causing severe problems, but you might explore CyberKnife as a means of eliminating them," he said.

Our conversation ended with some hope but little direction of finding a CyberKnife specialist. Dr. Sugarbaker did not recommend any specific hospital or doctor for this relatively new procedure. I am sure he did not want to endorse anyone with whom he did not have intimate contact. Finding a CyberKnife surgeon was the next step on The SMIK's list after consulting with Dr. Sugarbaker.

Dr. Lacy had told me about two Connecticut hospitals that had the CyberKnife machines, and they were my next two calls. Unfortunately, they had only done a total of fifty cases since acquiring the CyberKnife machine, none of which were in the liver. I wanted to go somewhere that had performed this procedure many times, as well as many times in that specific body part. I inquired if they knew any hospital that was better versed, and they both replied that they did not have that information. It was time to move up the CyberKnife chain of command.

Using the Internet, I found the corporation that makes the machine: Accuray, based in California.

"Accuray Corporation, how can I help you?" answered the pleasant woman on the other side of the country.

"Hello, this is Dr. Bob Rauch," I replied. "I would like to know if you can recommend the hospital that has performed the most CyberKnife procedures in the liver."

"I am sorry sir, but I do not have that information available," she responded cordially.

"I am sure that your statistics department would have some data on hospitals that do more procedures than others?" I continued.

"I am sorry sir, but we really do not usually share that type of information," she said as if to end the conversation.

This was not the time to be stopped. There was valuable information I needed and should be entitled to if I could get past her routine of "I am sorry … no."

"Let me rephrase the question," I said with courteous authority. "My name is Dr. Rauch, and I have a world-famous patient who needs CyberKnife surgery in the liver. He will go anywhere on the planet to get the best treatment. Unfortunately, I cannot divulge his name, but you would know who he is if I were to mention his name. All I am asking is, if you would please connect me with someone in your organization that might be able to recommend a hospital for my patient."

She hesitated, and then said she would check with her supervisor. I gave her my office telephone number and thanked her in advance for her kindness.

I was flirting with bravado and inappropriate behavior by somewhat misrepresenting who I was and who my patient was. I am a dentist and my patient was me. Even though I am not "world-famous," I do have friends all over the world. These were not lies, but truths clouded in shades of gray.

"Hello, Dr. Rauch's office, how may I help you?" Paulette, my office manager, answered the phone.

"I am from the Accuray Corporation in California and I have a list of numbers for Dr. Rauch."

"What is this in reference to?" Paulette asked attempting to avoid unsolicited cold-callers who try to sell me things.

"Dr. Rauch called me up and told me that he had a patient who needed CyberKnife surgery. I have the hospitals that are the recommended ones for his particular patient," the Accuray secretary responded.

Paulette took the numbers and smiled. She has been with me for over 20 years and has handled some unique calls without getting flustered. This was one of those calls. She tracked me down at lunch and I told her the story and thanked her for the numbers. It was time to move on down the list to the next task toward getting my cancer handled.

The recommended hospitals were located in Baltimore, Minneapolis, Miami, and Long Island. In less than two days, I connected with the secretary of each hospital that was in charge of the CyberKnife unit and asked them to be on the lookout for a package I would be sending them within a week. The next day, I put together four packets which included my CT scan; lab reports form recent blood tests, surgery reports and a copy of my first book. They were FedEx'd and would be at the hospitals within two days. Another step was crossed off of the list The SMIK and I had developed less than a week before.

Each doctor had a slightly different viewpoint concerning my case. That was somewhat disturbing, but unfortunately cancer is not like a math equation and there is no exact right or wrong answer. I knew that, but continued to talk with the CyberKnife doctors in order to figure out what they agreed upon before making my own decision on whether to proceed with CyberKnife, and which doctor I might use.

The last doctor I connected with was Dr. B. in Baltimore. We talked for almost an hour and he seemed extremely optimistic. Optimism in itself is not always a selling point. I have known many people who talk a great game but strike out all the time. This guy not only told me he had done over 1,200 CyberKnife procedures and had performed over 50 of them in the liver area, but he believed my case was very manageable with his technology. Our conversation was drawing to an end when he commented about my being an older man.

"I am only 58 years old," I said affronted by his inference.

"You were born on September 16, 1950: two days before me," he said humorously. "And I might have ethical problems operating on you because of your affiliation with the Yankees," he continued, throwing another humorous point that told me that he knew who I was as a person. He had read my book and was referencing information he had gleaned from it.

I had also done my homework on him and knew that he had gone to Tufts undergraduate and Harvard Medical School.

"If it takes me rooting for the Red Sox to have you save my life, I guess I will have to get myself a new hat tomorrow," I replied.

We ended our conversation with more than a doctor-patient relationship. "You will not die on my watch," he said as we shook hands. His words gave me hope and confidence that the new cancer spots on my liver would be eliminated and added conviction to my belief that he was the man I wanted to handle my case.

Two weeks later, Diana and I sat in Dr. B.'s office in Maryland and talked about the CyberKnife procedure. It is an amazing technological breakthrough in medical science and rather than going into the details, I recommend you Google "CyberKnife" and see what it involves.

At the end of the consultation, I reached into Diana's purse and withdrew an official Boston Red Sox hat and handed it to him. He was visibly moved by my gesture, laughed, and then hugged me and Diana.

"You will not die on my watch," he said once again, earnestly looking me squarely in the eyes.

"You had better plan on living a long time," I responded

In October of 2009 (four months after CyberKnife), my blood work showed that the cancer tumor markers were decreasing significantly. The CyberKnife surgery had destroyed the cancer cells that had been inaccessible to conventional surgery and chemotherapy.

In response, I sent Dr. B. a package that month with the following note:

I have good news and bad news. The good news is that my tumor markers have decreased considerably, giving evidence of the success of CyberKnife. The bad news is that you might want to try on the enclosed shirt so you will have somebody to root for during the World Series.

Inside the package was a Derek Jeter Yankees shirt. The Yankees were playing in the World Series; the Red Sox were not.

Lessons:

Do not stop searching for a solution or cure for your problem. You need to look and explore all possibilities, and never take no for an answer. Be courteous, creative and persistent.

New technology is being developed every day. You and your doctor should research all possible options before choosing a direction.

Your doctor is a professional person and deserves your respect. He or she is also a person with emotions and a sense of humor. Your relationship with your doctor and his staff should be more than purely medical. This might be one of the most important relationships you will have and it should not be "just about your disease." When Dr. B.

received the package, he called me up. "That was the best thing I have ever gotten. My wife and I laughed so hard," he said.

I don't think he actually wore the shirt, but I know that I made him smile and I will hold him to his promise.

PART TWO

STORIES AND LESSONS BEFORE CANCER

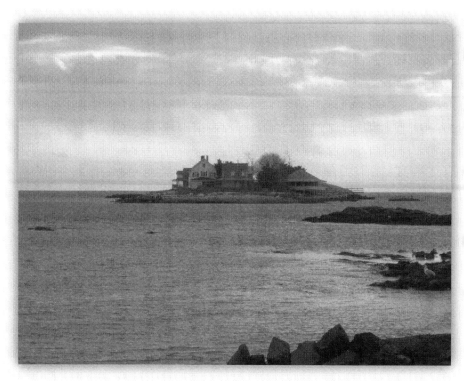

A home on one of the Thimble Islands

Another Angel

Branford is home to some of the most beautiful coastline Connecticut has to offer. About a mile away from Indian Neck in Branford, where my friend Ira lived, lay the Thimble Islands: a rocky outcropping of small islands and even smaller shoals that can barely be seen above the water. Large and small vessels alike have difficulty navigating.

Ira had recently purchased an abused, worn-out Aqua Cat at a tag sale. This boat was like a Hobie Cat, but a lot less expensive and a lot less sea-worthy. His Aqua Cat's 10 square feet of canvas netting stretched between two 12-foot pontoons and was connected to a stained and tattered sail. As the humble craft carried us up and down the coastline in front of Ira's home, it maneuvered like an old lumbering cow changing direction only if it desired to do so. The rubber gaskets around the pontoons looked progressively weaker each time we brought the boat ashore. We ignored the water draining from the supposedly airtight floatation devices and usually closed our sailing day with beer and steamed clams.

Friendships are formed in many ways, and my friendship with Ira began the year I graduated from dental school –1976– while I was single and working for Dr. Bednar in Derby, Connecticut. An orthodontist who was working in Dr. Bednar's building and knew both of us introduced me to Ira. He knew that Ira had also just graduated from dental school, and Ira and I had similar interests. A strong bond was easily formed between Ira and me that still connect us as brothers to this day.

One late September afternoon at about two o'clock, Ira and I hopped aboard the craft and headed out for a short sail. We had done this many times during the summer, but today we seemed to be in the mood for more adventure than the typical up-and-down-the-coast cruise. The wind was strong and directed us toward the Thimble Islands about a mile and a half away. We let the wind guide us as we traveled away from the protected shoreline, assuming we would get back before sunset. The clouds in the distance and the fog that was inoffensively rolling inland did not concern us. We sailed with the wind and would be at the Thimbles shortly. Any sailor (or anyone who was *thinking*) would realize the return trip would be against the wind and tacking (zigzagging) homeward would take us considerably longer than the trip there.

The wind quickened and our pace toward the Thimbles did the same. Unfortunately, one of the gaskets began to peel off and whatever ten cent glue might have been holding it allowed it to strip even more, leaving a white tail about four feet long running behind our craft. Thoughts of sharks looking at our dragging tail as if it were bait entered my mind, leaving me with concern and encroaching fear. If there were any sharks in the area, they were probably sand sharks and would not be of any life-threatening size. However, Spielberg's *Jaws* had left its mark: the image of monster sharks eating people in flimsy crafts flickered on and off in my head.

We were beginning to list as the pontoon with the peeling gasket seemed to be settling deeper and deeper into the water. The wind and darkening clouds were now coming in even quicker.

At this point, Ira and I decided we should probably turn around. However, the dilapidated Aqua Cat didn't respond to our urging and brought us further out to sea rather than closer to safety. The small emergency paddle Ira kept on board was of minimal use in turning the boat around as the craft fixedly lumbered out to sea.

It was an absurd moment, watching this silly little boat heading away from the mainland and now away from the Thimble Islands. Our ability to control the sail had become nonexistent. By now, the starboard pontoon which had been dragging the rubber gasket was half underwater and Ira joined it, by falling overboard in an attempt to reach and drag the gasket back on the craft. Rather than cling to the boat, he took a stroke and ended up on a rocky outcrop no bigger than his body. Other jagged rocks surrounded Ira's perch, threatening just barely below the churning water.

Then I tried to paddle close enough so Ira could jump towards the boat. The wind whipped the sail left and right. I wasn't sailing this boat – I was just trying to paddle it. Darkness began to descend and mist blanketed the choppy water. *Ridiculous*, I thought. It was getting cold, this boat was not sea worthy, we were in the middle of nowhere and no one even knew we were there. Some adventure.

It was now about five o'clock in the evening. The setting sun was barely visible through the darkening clouds and rain was beginning to fall. I tried three times to get close enough to Ira so he could jump onto the boat. The tide was coming in and Ira's rock would soon be totally underwater. Sharks again enter my mind. A great white was probably not waiting for dinner, but at this point, anything was possible.

Now I was afraid. Mother Nature was more powerful than I had ever seen. Her wind lapped the water causing waves to crash over the boat. The sail was flapping aimlessly in the wind, and the leaking pontoon was almost fully underwater. The best I thought I could do was to somehow run the ship aground on Ira's rocks and hope someone would find us the next day – if we were able to survive the night without sharks feasting upon us. We had angered the Sea Gods by traveling out on the silly Aqua Cat where good judgment should have persuaded us otherwise.

Finally, Ira and I were within five feet of each other. In a jump plus a few strokes he came on board, leaving us to drift away from what – in my mind– might have been a reasonable place to plant ourselves for the evening. We could not control the Aqua Cat, and in the dark fog we had no idea which way was home. We stared into the fog that had rolled in to the point where we could not see five feet in front of us. The wind grew stronger and the rain began to pelt us with considerable force. We sat in silence, our eyes terrified.

"I'll throw you a rope," a voice echoed in the near-darkness.

"What?"

"I'll throw you a rope. Catch it and hold on," the voice seemed to come from the middle of the wind. We looked behind us and saw a man with a white beard in a yellow raincoat and a yellow rain hat aboard a 20-foot-long Boston Whaler. He tossed us a line from the back of his boat which we grabbed with elation. We wrapped it around the lower part of our mast and held it with our hands. Slowly, he revved the engine forward and when the rope pulled taut he increased his speed so that we trailed behind him. About twenty minutes later, the shore line came into view.

When we were close enough to shore, the man backed off his engine so we could jump off and drag the half-sunken Aqua Cat to safety. We untied his rope and threw it back to him. He waved, smiled and turned his craft back to sea.

"Thank you!" we yelled as he faded into the mist. We beached the Aqua Cat, dragging it on shore as much as we could. It was incredibly heavy since one of the pontoons was filled with water. We collapsed on the beach, cold, wet, tired and in awe of the turn of events.

A man in a yellow rain coat rescued us from potential disaster. We giggled nervously and then broke into a guttural laughter, putting our arms around each other and letting the rain drip down our faces. The man had towed us to Stony Creek, which was about a 10-mile drive from Ira's home. We called Ira's roommate from a nearby bar and she came to pick us up in our soaked but smiling state. We left the Aqua Cat where it lay, not worried if it would still be there in the morning.

On the way back to his house, we told his roommate that we had met an angel.

Lessons:

Sometimes angels wear yellow hats and yellow raincoats.

"Thank you" is the appropriate response for an angel's help.

Angels show up at just the right time. You may think they should have shown up sooner, but sometimes your lesson is not yet finished.

If an angel throws you a rope, take it.

Mr. Woods: The Prophet

In 1981, Diana and I traveled to St. Thomas in the Virgin Islands for a beach vacation. We had been married two years, started a dental practice, moved to a new town and were pretty stressed out. This vacation was intended to rekindle the relationship daily life had clouded over.

The second day we were there, we decided to venture into town and called for a taxi. The local island taxi driver beamed with a smile that made you smile right back.

"Hello, my name is Mr. Woods." he bellowed.

His deep, bass range voice rang with a pronounced island twang. He had very dark black skin and graying hair. Gold glistened from several teeth. He seemed to be in his late seventies but carried himself like a younger man.

"Where do ya want ta go today, nice people?" he asked as he began to drive out of the hotel driveway.

"Downtown, please," I said.

"Very well, I will take you to my cousin's store and you can start there."

Local people promoting their relatives, I thought, skeptically, and begrudgingly accepted his starting point. My own in-charge attitude succumbed to Mr. Woods, but I felt somewhat uneasy being told where to go. Then again, we did not know where we wanted to go anyway and as long as he was taking us into town, anywhere would be a good place to start.

The ride was interesting. Mr. Woods waved to just about every taxi we passed, as well as many locals who happened to be by the side of the road. After every wave, he commented as to who the person was, including their name and relationship to him: cousin, brother-in-law, godson, grandson or nephew. And everyone he waved to waved back with enthusiasm.

"Here we are," he said as he dropped us off at a jewelry store smack in the middle of the business district. He told us the name of his cousin who worked there and proceeded to tell us what time he would pick us up that evening from the hotel.

"You should have no trouble getting a cab back to your residence after shopping, and I will pick you up tonight at seven and take you to a fine island restaurant," Mr. Woods said.

Who was this guy? I thought. *He's rather pushy and presumptuous.* Once again, I succumbed to his instructions. Our hotel was off the beaten path and getting a cab might have been difficult at dinnertime. Some restaurants had been recommended to us, but for one night, I guessed we could follow the local's suggestion.

"Thanks," I responded halfheartedly.

The shopping day was fun and we easily got a cab back with enough time to enjoy the beach and relax before getting ready for dinner.

By seven o'clock, Diana and I were outside our door waiting for Mr. Woods. By ten-after-seven I began to get a little anxious. Would we miss our reservation? Did we have a reservation? What restaurant were we going to? Who was this cab driver that just came into our vacation and started orchestrating my day and night? Moments later, Mr. Woods' bright smile and pleasant "Good evening, nice people," caught our attention.

During the ride to whatever restaurant he was taking us to, he seemed to be aware that I was checking my watch and feeling pressed for time.

"You know," he began, "too many people go through life rushing and hurrying and never smelling the roses. You should be patient today so you do not be a patient in the hospital tomorrow." After saying that, he let us out in front of a quaint restaurant with a beautiful view of the sea.

"I will be here for you at the end of the evening to take you home. Enjoy your dinner." With that, he drove away.

The hostess welcomed us as if we were stepping off the red carpet and greeted us like royalty. The manager was Mr. Woods' nephew and it seemed like everyone in the restaurant knew him or was related to him in some way. The meal was spectacular, the price almost too reasonable and the service four-star.

Our dinner conversation revolved around Mr. Woods' sage words concerning patience, how our lives were too impatient and how we needed to slow down our current pace to avoid future hospitalization. We laughed and wondered what words of wisdom he would have for us on the ride home. Sure enough, as we left the restaurant, there was Mr. Woods with his sparkling smile.

When he dropped us off at the hotel, he said, with his deep voice "I will pick you up tomorrow at nine in the morning and take you to a beautiful beach."

"Well," I responded, not wanting to be rude but not wanting to allow this man to totally control our vacation, "we may sleep late and just go to the pool tomorrow." It was a frail attempt to deflect his suggestion for the next day.

"No, you will like this beach. If you are not outside the door, I will know that you do not want to go. However, I am sure that I will see you tomorrow," he said, and then drove away.

"We could go to the beach tomorrow," Diana said.

"How do we even know where he is taking us?" I responded, somewhat frustrated.

"Has he led us wrong, yet?" she questioned.

"He took us to his cousin's restaurant!" I retorted, trying to make some obscure point directed towards distrust.

"It was a great meal!" Diana replied, pretty much ending the conversation.

Sure enough, at nine o'clock the next morning we were waiting at the door. And sure enough, Mr. Woods arrived at ten after nine.

"Good morning, nice people," he said with his ever-cheerful tone.

We entered the cab and once again almost every local we passed had a wave and a broad smile for our driver.

"Are you related to everyone on the island?" I asked chidingly.

"Not everyone," he said.

Then he began a story of a man and a woman: The man sees his wife aging and because the man only sees the outer beauty, he changes wives and goes with a younger woman. The man then sees his new woman aging and changes wives again. In the end of the story, the man has many alimony payments and three old women.

"If the man would have been smart," Mr. Woods stated, "he would have worked out his differences with his first wife and seen her for the beautiful girl he originally married." Then he dropped us off at a magnificent beach and told us he would pick us up at four o'clock.

I cannot recollect a more wonderful beach day. Not surprisingly, our conversation for most of the day revolved around Mr. Woods' new pearls of wisdom concerning wives and relationships. We discussed other peoples' relationships and our own. We knew people who went through troubled times and divorce seemed to be the typical answer. By the end of the day, our discussions ended on an incredibly high note. Even though we had normal marital issues, we were committed to our relationship and would work out any difficulties we might encounter in the future as well as handle the few that faced us now.

Just when we were ready to head back to our hotel, Mr. Woods appeared. He had just arrived and was waving to us from the road. We packed up our beach paraphernalia and walked the hundred yards over the soft, bleach-white sand to our self-appointed driver.

"Hello, nice people. Did you enjoy your day?" he asked

"Yes, very much," Diana and I responded.

The ride back was a total learning experience. He pointed out trees and the lines of mud that traveled the length of the trunk. He got out of the car and tapped a hole into one of the mud lines. Hundreds of termites scurried out of the opening and began to patch up the newly made defect.

"Nature is amazing," he began as we got back into the car. He continued his monologue with how God has plans. Everything happens for reasons and all God's creatures are important, even the termites. Before we knew it, we were back at the hotel and somewhat disappointed the oration was over.

Surprisingly, he did not even mention when he would pick us up or further arrange any of our time on the island. We were to be left on our own and go back to our own agenda.

The next few days were fun, but we missed our Mr. Woods. We discussed his comments and admired his attitude. Here was a cab driver who seemed to be happier than anyone we had ever met. Nothing seemed important to him except making others happy and sharing his warmth and love with anyone he came in contact with.

As fate would have it, the cab driver for our trip to the airport at the end of our vacation was none other than Mr. Woods.

"Hello, nice people," he said enthusiastically as we entered the cab with our own smiles, awaiting our parting philosophic words from the cabbie prophet. Sure enough, it did not take long between his waves to cars and people we passed until he dropped the ultimate life lesson upon us.

"You know the secret to a healthy marriage?" he asked. He then answered his own question without waiting for our response:

"Love." "Love is like a well of water that can be full or empty. If you take and take from the well of love, the well runs dry. If you give and give, then the well of love overflows and pours all over you. So you be good to her and she will be good to you. It is that simple."

We exited the cab and thanked him for his part in our trip. He probably doesn't know what an impact he made on our marriage and our lives. Since that time we will often recite "Woodsisms" whenever we loose sight of what is really important.

Six years later, we went back to St. Thomas. Our marriage was on very solid footing, the dental practice was growing strong and we were in great states of mind. This was a special island with a special meaning for us.

After settling in and spending some time at the pool we showered and prepared for dinner.

"Let's go to that restaurant where Mr. Woods took us," Diana said.

"Fine, let's see if the cab company knows Mr. Woods and see if he can take us there," I responded.

Then I called the taxi cab number from our hotel, asked if they knew Mr. Woods, and if he could pick us up. Sure enough, they knew him and they would see if he could be our driver for the evening.

Unfortunately, when the taxi arrived, it was not him. Our driver knew Mr. Woods and said he would let him know some people were asking about him and they would like to see him before they left the island.

Every time I called for a cab that week, I requested Mr. Woods and, much to our disappointment, he never came. Almost every driver knew him and responded like the first by telling us he would let Mr. Woods know we were looking for him.

Finally, as we were waiting for our cab to take us to the airport at the end of our vacation, a smiling driver pulled up in front of us. He was ten minutes late.

"Hello, nice people" Mr. Woods bellowed.

I am pretty sure he did not remember us, or have any clue how much his words strengthened our marriage and added to our individual lives. He was happy we remembered him, and that was good enough for us.

We loaded up our luggage and hopped into the back seat awaiting philosophical words from Mr. Woods: there were none.

We never saw him again, but he will forever be an integral part of our lives and his words will always be guide posts to keep us walking on solid ground.

Lessons:

If you choose a path and are not prepared to alter it, you may lose out on some valuable direction. There are sources and people you may never have thought could teach you anything but, trust me, they can.

If someone gives you advice and it makes sense allow your thought pattern some variety and give their suggestion a try. Being stuck in your "rightness" limits your ability to see other views and may limit your spiritual growth.

Once you have experienced something that helps you through life, you should share it with others by living the lessons you have learned. You do not need to overpower people to share the lessons you have experienced; just lead by example and others will be inclined to follow your path much to their benefit.

Sometimes a prophet can share a message; and once that message is gifted, the prophet can become just a nice man with a big smile and a deep booming voice driving a cab in St Thomas.

Goal setting

It's difficult to say "no" to Roger. It could be his persuasive logic or his persistence, but more likely than anything it's the promise that if Roger has an idea there's usually some major adventure to follow. We have known each other since freshman year in dental school where we met in lab No. 4. If your last name began with Q, R, S or T you were stationed in lab No. 4 for the next two years of your life.

I sat next to Richard Reddy, Roger Reckis and Mike Rotter, the grouping of which would quickly be known as the "4R's." To this day we are as close as any friends can be, and any two of us together is a recipe for a memorable experience.

This particular episode with Roger occurred in 1985, nine years after graduating dental school. Our life paths were similar in that we were married, each had two children, large mortgages on our homes and offices, and considerable personal debt and we were working hard just to keep our financial lifeboats afloat. There was no doubt that we were out-stretched economically and would often compare notes with little clue as to how we would become solvent.

"Bob, I've got a great idea," Roger said during one of our weekly phone conversations. A cold chill went up my spine and the hairs on the back of my neck stood erect.

"There's a course near you in Stamford, Connecticut, and we can come down for the weekend. It's a management company that guarantees to help us handle the financial hole we have both gotten into." A weekend with Roger, his wife Jill, and Diana at a hotel in Stamford, taking courses during the day and partying at night seemed like the perfect way to spend another $1,000 and pile more debt atop the mountain of money we already owed. The course was secondary to the party, and the plan sounded great.

We arrived Friday evening for the weekend course and partied all night with Roger and Jill. We still managed to get up early enough for third row seats in the filled conference room the next morning. There were over one hundred professionals (some with spouses) taking the course in similar hopes of obtaining financial stability. There I sat, with Roger on my left, Jill to his left and Diana to my right, pens in hand, course books in front of us, ready to learn.

Greg Stanley, the owner of Whitehall Management, stood at the podium finely dressed, looking sharp and confident as though he had the answers to solve everyone's problems. His business was flourishing, as he was a very well-spoken and intelligent economic guru.

As all good lecturers do, he began by engaging the audience with a simple question.

"How many here owe $25,000 or more? Raise your hands." Most of the audience raised their hands, including Roger and I.

"How many of you owe $50,000? $75,000? $100,000 or more? Keep your hands up." Many hands were still up at this point, but you could see where he was headed as the hands in the audience slowly started to drop.

"$200,000? $250,000? $300,000?" By the time he reached $400,000 in debt, the only remaining raised hands belonged to Roger and me.

Our wives sat beside us trying to bury their heads as they writhed with embarrassment. Both Roger and I withheld the desire to burst out laughing as we realized ours were the only two hands remaining high in the air. It's not often when a speaker looks directly at you in the audience and acknowledges your presence. Without further questioning of our indebtedness, he looked at us and said, "You can put your hands down." At which point Roger and I instinctively gave each other a high-five assuming we had won some grand acknowledgement.

"I do not believe that I can help the two of you," Greg Stanley said. "If you would like, I will refund your money." The statement seemed so hilarious at eight o'clock in the morning that we could barely contain our chuckles.

"Can we go to the bar now, Bob?" Roger whispered behind his falling hand.

"I guess so," I responded chidingly.

At that moment the tug on my shirt was sharp, as Diana's nails nearly ripped into the skin through my sleeve. Jill's reaction was similar.

Like little children reprimanded by their mother, Roger and I suppressed our mirth.

I do believe Greg Stanley was serious about refunding our money. The smirks left our faces as we looked from our wives back to the podium. We shook our heads, and refused. Then we directed our faces down to the desk, and Greg Stanley passed over us to continue with his lecture.

That was a painful weekend as I anguished over my financial stupidity all day Saturday and until the course ended Sunday at noon. Diana and I were financially doomed because debt would weigh us down for the rest of our lives. Often, Greg Stanley looked at Roger and me and used us as examples of what **not** to do.

I hated parting from Roger as I got into the car to drive Diana back home on Sunday. He was my only source for a potential smile and I knew the drive home would be filled with, "You should have!" "I can't believe you!" and "How could you have…?"

Rather than going directly home, Diana and I decided to stop at The Gathering, a restaurant in Milford, where we discussed the course lessons as they related to our future. Diana was, needless to say, disappointed with the likely outcome of our lives as Greg Stanley had pictured it.

Utilizing objective target setting techniques, I wrote down some goals for the next five years on the back of a business card and presented them to Diana before dessert. There was no attached plan to accomplish the goals, but just by writing them down I envisioned their fulfillment. A date was set to have these goals accomplished: 1990. I asked Diana to sign this little card, which she begrudgingly did to end the conversation, surely not believing a word I had written. The goals included a dental practice that grossed enough to pay off our debt within five years, a fully furnished home, cash in the bank, a published book and a *happy and mellow me.*

That night before going to bed, I placed that little card on my night table beneath the glass cover. Every morning I would turn off my alarm and look at that card. Every night when I checked my alarm before going to bed, I would look at the little card again. I had set these goals for myself and by reading them every day and night; I confirmed my commitment to attain them.

Five years later, to the date, I took out the card and took Diana to The Gathering for dinner. We had achieved everything on the list and more. We lifted our wine glasses and toasted the future.

Lessons:

A man of great stature had said we were doomed. My economic incompetence had destroyed us, and we might as well give up our dreams and aspirations of a bountiful life. I refused to believe that I was a failure at the age of 35 and further refused to believe that I could not achieve anything I wanted.

By writing goals down on paper, directing my energy toward accomplishing those goals and using some solid and sound business and financial techniques, I was able to accomplish all I set out to do.

Professional economic counsel is usually good advice to follow, however, blanket "across the board" recommendations **do not** and **should not** apply to everyone's situation.

Being in debt is not a good thing and should be avoided.

In my particular case, I had just bought a home, finished refurbishing another home for my dental practice and equipped it with state-of-the-art technology that allowed me to perform a high quality of dental care. Both investments would pay off in time as long as I worked hard and diligently to get out of debt as soon as I could.

Believe in yourself, believe that you can do anything and no one, no matter how intelligent they are, or how many credentials they have, can tell you that you can't.

Write down your goals, set your mind to them and achieve anything you want to.

Henry Ford said, "If you think you can or can't, you're right." **He was right**.

Route 17

On Christmas Day, 1980, Diana and I drove to Liberty, N. Y. to spend a long weekend with my parents. We would be meeting them that evening, staying in Monticello, New York, and would be skiing the other days at a little place called the Pines Hotel. I figured we would get an extra day skiing on Thursday at a different mountain before meeting my parents that night.

Diana and I went to Holiday Mountain and when we got there we were hesitant to ski because it was bitter cold. The temperature was as low as -6.9 degrees Fahrenheit, the wind was gusting up to 48.33 miles per hour and the wind chill calculation made the apparent temperature -41°F. At that temperature, frostbite can occur within ten minutes if a body part is not fully covered. It also appeared as though we would be the only ones on the mountain, as it was Christmas Day.

After two or three runs, we decided to call it a day, so we went to Monticello and checked into the hotel early.

The weekend was pleasant enough and because the weather was so bitter cold, we all decided skiing would not be appropriate. We shopped, enjoyed the small pool and had a relaxing weekend with my parents. Sunday morning was still bitter cold, and the breakfast waitress warned us to be careful of the treacherous icy roads for our return trip home. My overcautious parents requested we follow them down Route 17, after which my dad would head towards Brooklyn and I would cut over to Connecticut. Begrudgingly, I agreed, even though I knew he would be driving incredibly slowly and I could make much better time if I did not follow him.

We started down Route 17 from Monticello and my Datsun 280Z (my third one, having totaled my two others) was discouraged at having to follow Dad's Buick Riviera. It was not in my nature to go the same pace as my dad, but to keep my parents unstressed after my dad's warning; I decided to stay behind them.

The conditions were actually very bad. Route 17 freezes and I mean really freezes. The road had become an actual sheet of ice and it didn't take long before we were only going 10 miles per hour and I could feel the road slipping underneath me. I knew how easily it spun out of control. So the precautionary measure of staying behind my dad ceased to not annoy me.

I must have counted at least 20 cars that passed us early that Sunday as we drove home. Most of them were the new generation of four-wheel drive cars, station wagons or vans. A mile or two down the road, we passed these same cars that had slid off the road into the median strip or the side guardrail. It was the most treacherous ride I had ever experienced. Cars off to the left and right side of the road had gone too fast. My fear at this point was not that I would slip off the road, because I was actually going so slowly, but that other cars would lose control and bang into Diana and me or my parents.

It was a welcome sight when I saw the flares and policemen directing everyone off Route 17. I got off the exit as slowly as I could and followed my dad's car and the ones in front of him onto a small local road that headed south parallel to the highway. This road was also frozen. Everyone now should have been going 10 miles per hour because the line of traffic allowed them little alternative.

Unfortunately, American drivers hate being in traffic and even with hazardous conditions their driving patterns ignore the dangers. Many of the SUV yahoos who had not already skidded out were trying to pass everyone and move along faster than they should. Once again, I feared that they would skid into my car.

At that point, my dad and mom were several cars ahead of us and couldn't even see us. "Pull out the map Diana ..." I requested. It didn't take her long to find a road that headed north, even though we wanted to head south. My theory was that everyone was heading south and if we headed north for a short while, we could soon find another road that headed southeast, and thereby avoid this congestion. It was a brilliant and flawless philosophy ... so I thought.

At the next intersection, we took a left and headed north, leaving the traffic and the crazy drivers behind. Diana then found a little "red" road several miles ahead that would take us east and eventually put us back on to a main road on the other side of the Hudson River where we could continue our southeastward journey home to Connecticut. One summer day I'll go back to this little red road and see the beautiful scenery with a different perspective. However, this particular freezing winter Sunday morning the little red road that now would take us east would prove to be a life experience worthy of a chapter in this book.

We turned right with some minor concerns. The road headed uphill and there was icy snow on it because it had not been plowed recently. I found myself skidding a little bit, but as long as I kept the speed under 10 miles per hour, I was able to make the steady incline. To our left was an ascending sheer cliff that was growing larger with our forward progress. To our right was a guardrail that overlooked a similarly descending sheer cliff that ended about a billion feet below.

About fifteen minutes into this slow, steady climb, I fully realized that like a rollercoaster ride, anything that goes up must come down. Fear began to creep into every pore of my body. After a twenty minute climb, we reached what appeared to be the top of the hill. Panic struck me, but I don't believe Diana fully understood what was in store for us. She was too busy looking to the right and gripping her seat and praying. Our seat belts were buckled and reaching the crest of the rise, we began our downhill trek.

I never touched the gas pedal. No one was in front of me, and no one behind. It was obvious to me, at that moment, why no one else had shared my unique spirit of travel. I rode the brake, barely crawling down the mountain. The ice underneath us would not cooperate, and even at 2 miles per hour I could feel my tires slightly give way. I would ease off the brake just enough to allow the car to go straight then slightly ease down again hoping not to skid. I had both sides of the road on this mountain path to work with. There was no one ascending the hill, so even slightly skidding gave me enough room to the left and to the right. On our left side was a gully where the runoff from the mountain beside it would head downhill. Nothing was dripping, and the gully was full of snow: It was too cold for ice to melt. Fortunately, the guardrail to the right followed us all the way down the mountain. About fifteen minutes into the downhill journey, I had reached a speed of almost 20 miles per hour. I could not pressure the brakes much at this point without skidding and totally losing control.

It only took a second. I depressed the brakes ever so slightly and the car spun. It spun 180 degrees, before I managed to get back into control with another slight tap of the brakes. Now I was going down the hill backwards as if in a Burt Reynolds movie. I had pulled one of those spins like a stunt driver and was actually skidding backwards, looking in my rearview mirror and turning around while keeping my wheel as straight as I could. The braking and spinning had slowed me down to about 15 miles per hour, but I was going backwards and still way too fast.

Out of nowhere I looked uphill in front of me and saw a plow truck that was within 20 feet of us. I hadn't seen it before, probably because I had not looked in my rearview mirror since our descent began. Now I was looking straight at him and I could see fright and terror in his eyes. I can only imagine what he saw in mine.

He dropped his plow in order to slow himself down. Sparks flew from every corner of the metal plow blade as it dug through the ice and into the road. My car then veered sideways, so I tapped the brakes again for no reason in particular. At the same time, I gave a slight twist of the wheel, and the car spun around another 180 degrees. Now I was at least facing the correct direction. The plow truck had slowed down behind me, but I was using the whole road. I looked in front of me and I could not catch my breath before I saw a big yellow bus coming uphill.

You can't make this stuff up. It was amazing, as if I was in a dream. I don't think Diana was breathing at this point. Sheer terror covered her face. She was on the rollercoaster with me and neither of us could believe what was happening either. Fortunately for me, she wasn't grabbing me or yelling or doing anything at all but praying. Her prayers were probably the only logical thing occurring at that time.

The bus and I faced off. As best I could, I moved to the right side of the road. The bus driver's face had the same look as the plow guy's behind me: Terror. He moved a little to his right and the bus went into the ditch on the mountainside. Fortunately, he was going slow enough that there was no major damage to the bus or its passengers. They would be grounded until some huge tow truck could get them unstuck.

I guess they were driving home, or headed somewhere for the day and this would alter their journey and change their destiny. They would never go uphill and certainly never face the inevitable downhill slide. Luckily, their judgment would be enlightened and their path changed after our encounter. I shudder to think what would have happened had they reached the other side.

At this time the road began to flatten out and the ice beneath us became less slippery. The mountain cliff to our left disappeared and the railing to our right gave way to a road that entered into a little town. The plow truck behind us must have stopped near the bus because it was not in my rearview mirror any more. On the right was a shiny little diner and with no urging from Diana, I pulled in and stopped the car. My hands needed to be pried from the steering wheel, my elbows were locked in a straight position, and my breath was slow and shallow. Diana's eyes were wide open, her mouth agape. We looked at each other in sheer amazement as we got out of the car and walked into the diner, not saying a word. We sat at the counter and ordered two coffees.

It was one of those little towns where the diner was the local meeting place. Next to the cash register sat a CB radio where you could find out what was going on and the policemen could talk to the firemen and the truckers could talk to anybody. From that radio we heard a muffled voice,

"Ten-four, ten-four, a bus was run off mountain road by a little sports car. We've got plow trucks and tow trucks headed up. We believe the sports car was blue and headed east. Over."

"We'll have those coffees to go," I said.

The lady behind the counter poured them into Styrofoam cups, put lids on them and handed them to us. I put $2 on the countertop, and we got back into our blue sports car and headed home. The remainder of the ride was uneventful, and all we could do was repeat: "I can't believe it. I can't believe it."

We got home and my parents had called several times. They had made it home hours before we did.

Lessons:

I can read several spiritual messages from my experience on Route 17: Sometimes, you should stay on course. Don't go north when you want to go south. If the road is slippery go slow and try to avoid inclines because there is usually a downhill after the uphill.

I can also read a deeper message into the event: Sometimes you are just a cog in the wheel of others' lives and it is not about you. I believe Diana and I were being used to stop that bus filled with people from going up that hill. Had we not been there, that bus would have gone all the way up the hill and then it would have had to go down the other side and confront a similar experience to ours There is no doubt in my mind that no matter how good the bus driver's skill was, he could not have pulled two 180 degree turns and managed to stay on the road. The guardrail overlooking the cliff would not have held back a bus and the passengers would not have exited the event unscathed. Either I was a great driver, or somebody else was controlling my vehicle at that time. I saved those people in that bus by running them off the road. Our reward was a hot cup of coffee and a great story.

I sold that Datsun shortly after.

The Helmet

Thank God I was wearing a helmet when the Toyota Corolla slammed into me and my bicycle and thrust me into the windshield and over the roof, tossing me to the ground yards behind the vehicle. My bicycle, a beautiful black 27-speed, $1,500 Cannondale, lay mangled under the driver's front right tire and promised never to ride again. I was extremely fortunate to find a different fate than my bike that early spring morning in 2003.

Wendy, Rob and I had been biking together for almost 10 years. We usually leave my house at six in the morning for an hour-long, 13 mile ride along the Milford coastline. The early morning ride works on many levels for our schedules and psyches. The beauty of the rising sun, the waking wildlife and most importantly, the minimal traffic all impart a special flavor to our ride. The conversation transgresses from spiritual to smut within an hour, and our bodies as well as our souls ride a little stronger by the time we end.

This particular day was no different except for the last stop sign we approached. I was leading the others, cruising up the minor incline preparing to stop. Wendy and Rob were to my left and slowing down as well. We are seasoned riders and had plenty of close encounters with terrain hazards and those dreaded automobiles and their inconsiderate or distracted drivers. At this particular stop sign, I stopped, looked both ways and then proceeded as per the rules of the road. It was a four-way intersection with stop signs on all four corners, so I did not expect any moving traffic from either side of me as I entered the intersection.

Oh, how surprised I was when out of the corner of my right eye I saw the blur of a car blowing right through the stop sign. He was probably going about 30 miles per hour and never saw me in front of him. As I was barely moving, I had no momentum to dodge out of his way or direct my bike anywhere. The speed at which this happened also took any of my avoidance possibilities out of the equation.

I remember feeling my right side connect with his bumper as we made hard impact. Fortunately, at that instant my body's instincts took over control of my torso and limbs, instructing them to go with the flow of motion. Upon contact, my upper body twisted toward the car and my bike slid under its wheels. Then I felt my shoulder contact the hood, followed by the top of my head smashing against the windshield. The noise was as loud as a sledgehammer hitting a piece of sheet metal. My neck buckled and my body was flung over the roof of the car, which was now screeching as the driver slammed on the brakes.

The slowing motion of the car enabled me to bounce off the trunk before rolling on the asphalt for another 10 feet before coming to rest flat on my back.

The main impact had been between my helmet-covered head and the windshield. Throughout my acrobatic flying act, Rob and Wendy had their respective close encounters with this car. Fortunately, they had a moment and a few feet more reaction time to help them avoid my fate. Rob veered left and pulled up the front of his bike, slamming on his brakes and barely catching the front left bumper of the slowing vehicle.

He and his bike came out undamaged. Wendy slammed on her breaks and was able to avoid any contact at all.

My senses dulled the moment I realized what was happening; any physical pain would come after the ordeal ended. When I came to a stop, I looked skyward from the ground, assessing the damage.

There was little. I felt fine. Whatever contortions my body had gone through had enabled me to avoid any major bodily injury. The only thing that was broken was my bicycle and my helmet, which was cracked right down the middle.

Seconds after I recovered my total awareness, I saw Rob kneeling over me. Wendy was right behind him.

"Are you okay?! Are you okay?!" they yelled in a frantic chorus.

"I think I'm fine," I responded somewhat confidently.

Then the driver came running over, echoing Rob's statements. With his ashen-white face he looked as though he would have a heart attack on the spot if I did not stand to reassure him he had not killed me. I did just that, calming him down by proving that I could move. Rob, Wendy and the driver were amazed at my calm and compassionate attitude towards a man that had run me down moments before. Some force (God) had saved me, and anger was the last thing I wanted to display. The driver was more shaken than I, and I am sure God would not want me to berate this man any more than he already had done to himself.

I am not sure why I was "used" in this man's life, but I am sure there was some master plan that included me as part of the equation. The good news was that I came out undamaged. Obviously this man's day had been changed, as well as his view of driving and probably his view of life as well. That moment certainly affected my day and life, and I thank God for placing the helmet on my head that saved me.

You see, we had been riding for some time without helmets. In fact, I was the last in my group to don the plastic cap. That was one of my first morning rides with it on my head and I will never again ride without one.

Lessons:

Wear helmets when they are recommended – i.e. biking, skiing, baseball, etc.

If you are part of an accident, anger is not necessary. Your emotional response and finger-pointing will rarely improve the situation, and the fault and cause of the accident are not always obvious. Sometimes there is a bigger picture you may never know about.

It is not always favorable to be the lead rider. He is the most likely to encounter dangers.

The corollary to the previous thought relates to what is said at the Iditarod dogsled races in Alaska: "If you're not the lead dog, the scenery never changes."

Stop at stop signs and look both ways *carefully*. Then proceed with caution.

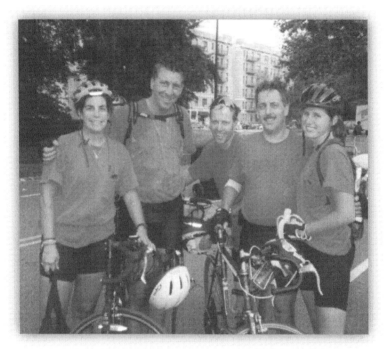

Team Orange members

Wendy, me (the captain), Sandy, Rob and Sarah

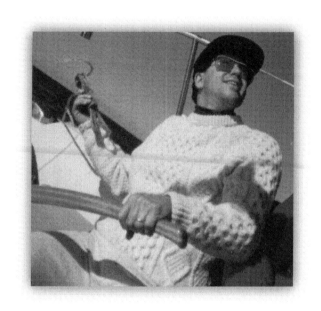

Jimmy holding torn dinghy rope

Smooth Sailing ... Not

Sailing is not usually dangerous. Obviously, a sailor must take necessary precautions to ensure that if problems arise, preparations are in place to secure the safety of those aboard. A more important step than being prepared for trouble is avoiding potential trouble in the first place. That was our first mistake.

Jim and I go on a sailing trip on Long Island Sound every year. Sometimes we go for a day trip and sometimes we go for a long weekend. Jim's boat is a 30-year-old 30-foot Catalina sloop. He maintains the boat well, but there is always something to fix during our voyage: the engine, the septic system, the anchor, and even the sail. This year, our trip would take us across the Sound and we would dock in Port Jefferson, Long Island, for the weekend and return Sunday night. Leaving Friday afternoon was imperative if we wanted to get across the Sound and meet up with Jim's brother-in-law, Neil, who would be there by seven o'clock that evening.

"What about those clouds over there?" I asked Jim, looking in a westerly direction at some ominous dark clouds as we were loading the boat with food and other supplies for the trip.

He looked out toward Long Island and waved his hand dismissing any worry of bad weather interfering with our three to four-hour journey. I assumed he had fully charted our course, consulted the weather reports and done all of the other necessary things on the pre-sailing checklist. He hadn't. This short trip was like walking from the bedroom into the kitchen for any sailor in the area. It was a straight shot and he had done this run before without any problems.

Jim leashed on his new dinghy, and looked at me smugly.

"I just bought this $2,000 dingy for your wife, Diana, you know."

Diana worried any time I went on trips with any of my guy friends, and worried even more when I went with Jimmy. He had a little blow-up life raft, but on our last trip Diana had insisted that in case of trouble it would not be enough. She made him promise to get a real survival craft or she would not let me travel with him. Obviously, he was a more prepared sailor with his new dinghy, but the fact that he could reference Diana as a reason for him spending money gave him some haughty pleasure.

He finished tying the dinghy to the back of the boat with a bright yellow, one-inch-thick 500-pound test nylon rope, then we hopped on board and left Milford harbor. He set the LORAN (the sophisticated guidance device), consulted the map, raised the two sails, confirmed that his radio was working and then pointed our boat in a southerly direction. With a sailboat, it is necessary to aim in the general direction you want to go, but to maximize your speed you need to harness the wind and redirect your craft along the way in order to get to your destination.

The wind was strong with occasional gusts that beckoned some creaks and groans from the fiberglass of the old craft. We were moving as fast as the boat had ever moved with the winds increasing every mile we traveled. Our joy overflowed. We were two good friends, talking and laughing about whatever the topic was, drinking some wine and feeling the power of the wind as we screamed across the surface of the water. The boat was leaning about as much as she could and the sails were bellowed out to their maximum. Water splashed over the side, which tilted nearly to sea level, and our backsides hung over the edge as real sailors do.

We had turned the motor off but left the key precariously positioned near the throttle. We would be in Port Jefferson long before our estimated time of arrival, and using the motor for power seemed ludicrous.

The first sign of problems began with some scattered clouds that were laden with rain. They came in waves and seemed to be random, but the intensity of the droplets stinging us was more than any usual rain. There were clear skies ahead and the weather moving in from the west did not seem like it would reach us before we got to Port Jefferson Harbor.

We had just passed the halfway mark when the pelting rain started to intensify. The winds were no longer coming from just one direction, the sails flapped inconsistently and our forward motion had come to a halt. I scanned in every direction and saw neither one boat nor piece of land. We seemed to be in the middle of a weather pattern that resembled the eye of a hurricane. Later we found out about the treacherous weather that occasionally flares up in the middle of Long

Island Sound. That would have been a good bit of information to have before we began our sail.

Unfortunately, – and much to the regret of our seamanship – both sails remained fully open, but now they were not even moving. An eerie calm settled in all around us.

"Jim, look at those clouds!" I said, looking due west.

Once again, Jim looked southward towards Port Jefferson. "There is a patch of blue and those clouds don't look so bad," he responded.

With more urgency in my tone, I pointed at the mass of clouds that was moving at a visibly intense speed towards us from the west. "Not those clouds. THOSE CLOUDS!" I exclaimed.

We both looked at this dark mass as it began to form into a funnel-shaped swirling torrent that was heading right for the side of our boat. The ominous cloud was about 100 yards away, and made it to our boat in a few seconds. We idled, frozen and there was little we could do to avoid it slamming into us. It was about 100 feet high from the water to its indiscriminate end in the dark, black sky. Like a locomotive thrusting forward into us, it lifted the back half of our boat in the air and pressed into the sails, forcing our 30-foot craft onto its side. The funnel cloud went through us effortlessly, as though we were light and fragile – like a matchstick. Jim was knocked down to the floor of the eight-foot-by-four-foot cockpit area. I held onto whatever I could grab and felt the water on my back as it rushed into the boat.

The boat was now totally on its side with water rushing into the cockpit and draining down into the lower part of the craft. The sails were underwater and kept the boat from righting itself. The large five-foot-long keel was beginning to elevate out of the water, and if it were to fully surface, the boat would surely turn upside-down and capsize, leaving Jim and me afloat for as long as we could swim. Did I mention that we were not wearing life preservers and that they were securely fastened below deck and inaccessible to us now?

The torrential rain began to waft over the scene, compounded by swirling winds which caused the sea to churn with three to five-foot swells. If there were any way to take a photograph of us at that moment, our faces would graphically display mixed emotions including, but not limited to: shock, awe, fear, amazement, terror, confusion, helplessness, and especially regret for being in this predicament in the first place. It would have been on the cover of *Time* magazine and the caption might have read: **Helpless men caught in Mother Nature's grasp.**

For those unfamiliar with sailboats, once the sails are in the proper position to catch the wind, the rope that moves the sail independently from the body of the boat is locked in place. The sheet, as it is called, is wedged into a device called a cleat that can be easily unfastened and repositioned when necessary. It was at this moment in time absolutely necessary to allow the sail to remain where it was by temporarily disengaging its connection with the ship, which was heading underwater. By releasing the sheet from the cleat, the boat should right itself, then the sail would slowly rise from its submerged position and drain the water that was dragging us down.

It was not my boat and I was not the captain or the one who should make the decisions. However, I did teach sailing on little one-man sailboats at a summer camp and had been on many other sailboats where I was educated on the basics of sailing. This was no time to stand on ceremony and ask Jim, who was on the floor, if it was all right to disengage the sheet. I tugged on the sheet and it did not release. Then I yanked with full force and the cleat released, leaving me with the sheet in my hand. Nothing happened for a second or two. Then, slowly, the boat began to lean to the upright position, followed by the flapping mainsail. The other sail, the jib, which was also underwater had less impact on our situation, but it followed suit and lifted out of the water as well.

The immediate peril had passed, but our present situation revealed flapping sails that needed to be lowered and a cockpit filled with water. Furthermore, the precariously placed key to the motor was missing, the LORAN and radio were shorted out and would not work, and we had been blown off course and did not know our exact position in relation to Port Jefferson. The integrity of the boat was suspect after such a violent hit and the wind-roughened sea and rain were intensifying.

Jim lowered the sails, I found the key to the motor and got it started, we checked with the compass and pointed the boat southward, and put on our life jackets and bailed out the water from the cockpit. I called 911 on my cell phone just to let someone know that there were two idiots somewhere in Long Island Sound.

I cannot quote any of the immediate conversation Jim and I had because the adjectives we used would not be appropriate for this text.

Suffice it to say we were amazed, blown away and totally in awe of what had just happened.

When we were done with our initial reactions, I looked at Jim and said, "I thought we were going under."

"I thought we were, too. But I knew that we would at least have the dinghy that Diana made me get if anything happened to the boat," Jim said confidently.

As he said that, he smiled and tugged on the bright yellow 500-pound test nylon rope that was connected to his new dinghy. There was no resistance. **There was no dinghy**. The rope had been torn during the maelstrom, setting the dinghy adrift. We never found it.

Concern mixed with laughter at that moment, but it was overshadowed by the sight of land. The buoy marker for Port Jefferson Harbor appeared out of the fog and rain less than a few- hundred yards away.

Before our return trip on Sunday, we checked with the Weather Channel.

Lessons:

Take nothing for granted. Smooth seas and clear skies can give way to disaster instantly with a single gust of wind.

Even when you are prepared with an extra lifeboat, realize it might not be there when you need it. There are stronger forces that laugh at meek attempts at preparation. However, those same powers can right your tipped boat as easily as knocking it down.

When you lose your direction, the natural laws of physics should always work. A magnetic compass can get you back on course, and a spiritual compass will never fail you.

Man's Best Friend

"Robert's. Duke of Seaview" was the official name of the puppy that sat on my lap as we headed home from the pet store. I was thirteen years old and the happiest kid on the planet. The eight-week-old Fox Terrier would be the best-trained, smartest and most loyal pet that anyone in my town of Seaview, Brooklyn, would ever have. NOT!

Duke was a typical small dog with a big attitude and no respect for authority. Unlike Lassie, the perfect dog of my generation, Duke was everything Lassie wasn't

He would not come if you called him, run away if he was not on a leash, and slept on the pillows rather than at the foot of the bed. He bit my cousin, Marty, while we were wrestling (we never told anyone), dug up most of my mom's flower plantings and chewed up many pieces of furniture. The "bad behavior" list goes on and on. Regardless of Duke's poor manners, he quickly became a family member and this boy's best friend.

He was there during my tough times as a youth, and his curly hair soaked up many of my tears. He went on family vacations and all but had his own seat at our dinner table. Duke was as much of a family member as Mom, Dad, or my brother, Howie. The only time Duke was separated from the family was for a week or two during the summer. Mom and Dad would take a vacation while Howie and I went to a sleep-away camp for eight weeks. During that time, Duke boarded at a pet store.

When I was twenty years old, I was a counselor in Nicholson, Pennsylvania, and Howie was working in Florida for IBM. My parents were vacationing in Europe, and Duke was boarded, once again, at the neighborhood pet store.

"Bob, there is a message for you at the main office," one of my co-counselors said.

At lunchtime, I retrieved the message that suggested I call my neighbor, Adrian, in Brooklyn. We had been living next to Adrian and her husband, Larry, and their two girls, who were similar in age to Howie and me, for at least 10 years. We were their emergency contact, and they were ours. I called her back immediately.

Adrian's voice was noticeably holding back emotion "Duke is very ill, and the man at the pet store is not sure what to do. He believes that your dog might not make it another day. You might want to come home," she said, knowing Duke was family.

Within 15 minutes, I packed a small bag with some necessities and was headed to my car ready for the three-hour drive home. I stopped into the director's office to tell him of my family emergency.

"You can't leave now!" he said with authority. "It is not your day off, and who is going to cover your duties at the waterfront?" I was the boating director as well as in charge of a bunk of eight children.

"My co-counselor said that he would cover the bunk, and the head of the waterfront said that they would cover my duties while I was gone," I said showing I had acted appropriately in arranging for my responsibilities to be handled in my absence.

"It's a dog, Bob," he said, inferring that my emotionally driven emergency was relatively unimportant and my running home was an over-reaction. He further alluded to the possibility that I might lose my job if I left without his approval.

"I am going home," I said as I left his office, willing to take whatever consequences followed. My Pontiac Firebird flew home, making the trip much quicker than the estimated three hours.

Entering the pet store was one of the saddest moments of my life. All of the dogs were yipping and barking and jumping around, while Duke lay motionless in an isolated cage in the corner of the room. After a brief discussion with the pet store owner, I exited his store with Duke draped over my arms. He was breathing with much effort. His eyes seemed to recognize me, but that was the only sign of life in my dog. The drive from the pet store to my home was less than 10 minutes, but it seemed as though I was heading nowhere and would never get there.

I entered my empty house, and then lay on my bed holding Duke, crying and asking God for help. Even though I was an intelligent person, knowing what to do during a crisis at a young inexperienced age was beyond my grasp. Hug, cry and pray for a miracle seemed to be my best solution to the situation.

The doorbell rang and jolted me out of my self-imposed stupor. Duke lay there, unmoved by the noise or my jumping out of bed. Adrian was at the door, and she hugged me, temporarily easing my grief.

"Bob, I called my veterinarian, and he suggested that we bring Duke to his office." With no further coaxing, Adrian drove me, with Duke in my lap, to the vet's office. After some discussion, we agreed leaving Duke there in an oxygen tent and hooked up to intravenous fluids as well as some other medications would be the best course of action to potentially save his life. When I finally returned home, I cried and prayed until I fell asleep after setting my alarm so I would be at the doctor's office as soon as it opened.

Duke was standing and barking and seemed to be his usual feisty self when I arrived the next morning.

"There are many possible reasons why Duke nearly died, but you can see that the treatment we performed worked. I recommend that Duke stay here several days until your parents return from vacation," the veterinarian said. He assured me Duke would be all right and I should return to my responsibilities at camp.

I thanked Adrian and the doctor, kissed Duke and headed back to Pennsylvania, ready to face the camp director's wrath. The long and arduous drive took more than three hours.

"I am sorry, so very sorry for my behavior," he began before I could say a word. "I did not understand the relationship between you and your pet. While you were gone, many campers and counselors educated me as to the relationship between 'family' members. I never had a pet, and I guess I missed out on a piece of life. I am sorry," he said.

He was so moved that I didn't even need to respond. Duke had become a camp icon and everyone's concern lifted my spirits even more than Adrian's daily calls acknowledging Duke was okay.

Lessons:

There is truth to the saying "A dog is a man's best friend."

Emotions can sometimes be your guide. Leaving camp and running home might not have been the smartest thing to do, but it turned out to be the right thing to do.

Not everyone can relate to the strong bond between a person and his pet but they might someday learn and become more whole as a person.

Prayer might bring an angel named Adrian knocking at your door to guide you when you are distraught and in need of guidance.

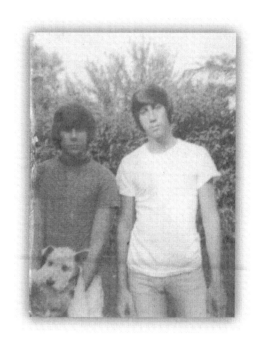

Duke, Howie and me

More Duke

Two summers later, I was working at a different camp in Copake, New York, as a camp counselor and boating instructor. The camp in Nicholson, Pennsylvania, was no longer in business. Andy, my college roommate, and I were co-counselors, and we were having a fantastic summer. Most days were spent relaxing at the waterfront directing the campers in boating skills and safety and teaching them the fine art of water fights. We filled the evenings with activities like camper talent shows, competitive games, and campfires.

Near the end of July, my folks went away on their traditional vacation. Fortunately for Duke, he was not boarded at the pet store. My brother, Howie, was home and would be watching over him and our home.

"Pull over the car," I said to Andy.

We were driving to town on our afternoon off, and just off the road I spotted one of those free-standing telephone, the kind that has a metal cover surrounding the black phone – a half phone booth, the kind that Superman would pass right by. The phone was at the beginning of a dirt road that led to an RV park. Copake is a beautiful resort area with camps, RV parks, state forests, lakes and mountains everywhere.

It was odd that I noticed the phone, because there was so many other things that should have captured my attention. The trees were all shades of green and in full bloom, the dark-blue sky was accented by white puffy clouds and Andy's stereo was blasting rock music as we sped down the back country road.

"What?" he responded?

"Pull over!"

Andy stopped the car, expecting to see a pretty girl hitchhiking or at least a scenic vista. When I exited the car, he understood why I asked him to stop. The one public phone at our camp was constantly in use by campers and counselors. There was a sign-up sheet for the prime calling hours – lunch and evenings. I had wanted to check in with Howie for the past several days and see how Duke was doing, but had been thwarted in my attempts to get phone time. Andy cranked up the stereo even more and rocked to the sound of Jethro Tull's "Locomotive Breath," as I walked to the phone.

As I picked up the receiver, a dog sauntered over to me from the edge of the woods. The man who appeared to be his owner stayed at the woods' edge in the shade of the large oak trees about fifty yards away. The man's grey hair sprouted in all directions under his baseball cap. His khaki shirt and shorts blended him into the surrounding trees, rendering him almost invisible. His walking stick gave him a Moses-like appearance, and it was obvious that he was an older man.

The dog was not nearly as old as the man, but did have the maturity and poise of an adult canine. I put the phone back on the hook and bent down to pet the dog, which was now standing politely at my feet. The man acknowledged my beaming smile as I started petting the dog. The coincidence was pretty powerful and unmistakable. The dog was a Fox Terrier with almost the exact coloring as my Duke. Keep in mind that Fox Terriers, especially wire-haired ones like Duke and this dog were not common. I had seen less than 10 of them my whole life, and here I was in the middle of nowhere with a well-behaved Fox Terrier befriending me.

After a few moments of petting my new friend, I stood up and picked up the black telephone and pressed it to my ear.

"This is the operator, how may I help you?"

"I'd like to make a collect call to 212-251-5935, please," I said.

While she was doing her dialing/connecting thing, I heard the man at the edge of the woods give a slight whistle. The dog perked up his ears, looked up at me – capturing my attention – then trotted to the trees and stood next to the man. They both stared at me, leaving a picture indelibly imbedded in my mind.

"Yes, I will accept the charges," Howie said on the other end.

My attention refocused on the phone and left the man and the Duke look-alike, who were now drifting into the woods like the mist disappearing when the sun rises on a foggy morning.

"Bob," Howie said somberly.

"Hey Howie, how are you doing and how is Duke?"

He hesitated, and then said words that crushed him and devastated me.

"Duke is dead."

Silence permeated everything. Neither of us spoke for an interminable minute or two. Tears rolled down my cheeks, and no energy was extended to stop them. Howie and I talked for a little while longer consoling each other. Mom and Dad would be home in a few days, and we decided Howie would tell them when they got home rather than share bad news during their short, worry-free vacation time.

I looked back to the woods as I hung up the phone and wiped my wet cheeks with the sleeve of my t-shirt. The man and the dog were gone. Had they ever really been there? The whole block of time since Andy stopped the car seemed out of step with what we consider reality. This was my first real confrontation with the death of a loved one. My grandmother had died years before, but that was different. I loved her and our blood-related family bond was strong, but my grandmother and I only spent hundreds of hours together. Duke and I had spent thousands.

The experience from two years before had alerted me to a future moment when Duke would die, so my shock at this moment was tempered. The fact that I had been gifted with a visit by a Duke look-alike and the grey-haired man further eased my pain. It did not take much imagination to believe Duke came to say goodbye to me.

Andy did all the right things a friend would do as I got into the car, obviously distressed. He listened to my tale and responded with compassion and remorse for my loss. On a curious note, Andy had not seen the man or the dog.

Lessons:

Phone home: Keep in touch with family and friends.

Having a pet can teach you so many things, but more often than not, it is a person's first experience with the painful loss of a loved one. The fish, the hamster, the cat and the dog are stepping stones for the future partings. I have lost my mother to cancer, my father to a heart attack, my brother, grandparents, aunts, uncles, father-in-law, brother-in-law, nephew and many friends. There can be no comparison of the loss of a pet and a person: They are apples and oranges. However, my ability to confront deaths of my family and friends as well as my own future demise has been greatly enabled by Duke's visit to me at the telephone booth in the woods.

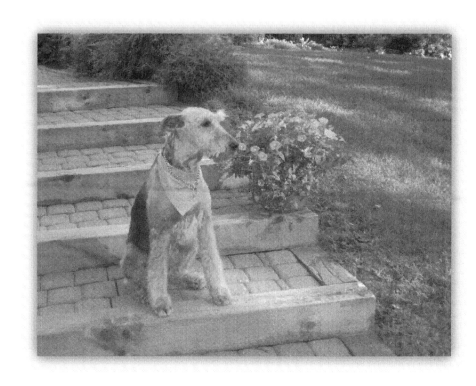

Duchess

Duchess

Our third child, Bryan, has a problem. Fortunately, I believe it will work to his advantage in dealing with life in his future. The word "no" does not compute in his world when the reasons for "no" are not practical, logical, fair and clearly spelled out.

"No," my wife Diana said to Bryan on his third birthday.

"But Mommy why can't I have a dog?" the little tyke asked Diana, standing up tall and looking her squarely in the eyes, waiting for an answer.

"Because."

"Because why?"

"Because I said so."

That conversation went on for three years – every birthday and every Christmas. In Diana's defense, she had some very good reasons for not wanting a dog. The primary reason was that she was afraid of them because of a childhood accident when her family dog had bit someone. Her personal fear and the fear of having a dog that might bite one of our children or their friends were real concerns. Second, she believed the associated extra work and dog "mess" would put her over the edge. As it was, she was already managing a very active household with three children, managing my dental practice and volunteering hundreds of hours at our children's schools and local community groups. She had no time or desire to add another life form to our family.

I understood her point, but still tried in vain for three years to convince her we could choose a breed of dog that would not bite children and not leave dog hair all over our home.

"No," Diana said.

"Why?" I asked after answering her concerns with logic and reason.

"Because," she said.

"Because why?" I responded

"Because I said so!" she said, ending our conversation for three years in a row.

The week leading up to Christmas during Bryan's sixth year of life was like an interpersonal chess game that included every family member taking strategic diplomatic positions interposed between Bryan and Diana: to dog or not to dog. No one wanted to stand up too strong to Diana, yet seeing how deep Bryan's desire for a dog was made it difficult not to take his side. This year, however, Bryan enlisted the support of a heavyweight: Santa Claus.

"Bryan," Diana said with some frustration, "What else do you want?" she was standing in our hallway holding Bryan's annual Christmas list. Bryan's list was short.

Bryan's Christmas List

A dog

"Bob, please talk to him," Diana said, handing me his list and leaving the room.

"Bryan, what else would you like Santa to get you?" I asked with a clearly defined mission.

"Daddy, I think I was good all year and Santa will get me what I want. If I put anything else on my list, he will probably get me the other stuff and not the dog, which is all I really want," he said.

His logic was flawless, and no matter how subtle I was, he would give no hint of desiring anything else but a dog. His sister, brother and grandparents could not dislodge any information either.

On Christmas Eve, Diana and I were wrapping gifts and checking off who got what and there was no avoiding Bryan's two-word list: but there was no dog to wrap. After hours of negotiations with Diana (when she was barely awake and worn out by wrapping), she gave in to a halfway measure. Bryan would receive a glitter-covered **gift certificate from Santa "You will get a dog in the springtime."**

I told Diana that Bryan would probably forget about the card, and by springtime his desire for a dog would have faded. We both knew that was improbable.

On Christmas day, the look of disappointment on Bryan's face was evident. His brother and sister opened their gifts wildly while Bryan opened his gifts sadly after realizing there was not a puppy with a ribbon around his neck under the tree. The heartbreak was palpable to the entire family and just before tears welled up on his little face, I handed him the envelope containing the gift certificate. He knew that it wasn't a puppy and all of the presents had been unwrapped. Begrudgingly, he opened it.

The glitter fell onto the carpet and the heavy colorful paper was firmly held between his hands. Slowly, he read the nine words that transformed tragedy to triumph: YOU WILL GET A DOG IN THE SPRINGTIME – SANTA. He read it again, connecting the words and the meaning of the sentence. I am sure you can imagine the relief and elation he felt. The only tough moment was when he walked over to Diana and read the words loud and clear with emphasis on "Santa," and enunciating with a 'humph,' to demonstrate the definitive power behind the forthcoming gift. Diana took it in stride and smiled as the wonderful mother she is. She would have to deal with her fears and accept the additional burdens because getting a dog was inevitable.

At Bryan's request, a calendar was placed in his room and the first day of spring was circled. There would be no way of postponing or avoiding the Dog, even though Diana and I never discussed it. I researched all possible breeds and chose the Airedale terrier as the breed of dog that would fit best with our family. The breed does not shed, is wonderful with children, loyal to families, obedient when trained well and usually a healthy dog if bred well. The only problem was finding that breed of dog. With limited computer technology and skills, it presented a challenge. When the time came, I would worry about how I would find one.

"How will Santa bring me the dog? … How will we know that it is the right dog? … How will we know the exact day when he will come? … What kind of dog will it be? … " Bryan asked. His daily questions were directed to me because he knew his mother would not be enthusiastic about any conversation regarding the Dog.

"There will be a sign," was my standard response.

"What kind of sign?"

"We will know it when we see it," I always said, fulfilling his need for an answer as well as giving myself some wiggle room as to the dog specifics.

The day of reckoning came sooner than I imagined.

"Dad, it's the first day of spring," Bryan said, standing in front of me holding the card from Santa while I sat at the kitchen table having a cup of coffee. "Am I getting my dog today?"

Now if this were a movie, picture the scene. It was the day before Easter Sunday. Diana had left to go to the grocery store. The newspaper – that I never read – was strewn on the table in front of me where Diana had left it after pirating some coupons. The portable telephone was on the table in front of me – left there from Diana's earlier conversation, and Bryan stood there with unbridled enthusiasm ready for the fulfillment of a dream ready to come true.

Avoiding his eyes, I looked down at the table toward the newspaper. And it read "**Dogs for sale,**" Airedales were the first breed on the alphabetically organized list. Putting my coffee down, my hand moved two inches and I replaced the cup with the phone.

"Can I help you?" asked the male voice.

"Do you have Airedale terrier puppies for sale?"

"Yes, I have one left."

Lessons:

Duchess has been a member of our family since that day, and even though Diana and Duchess had strained relations at the beginning, they are best friends now. I do not mean best friends in just the typical "man's best friend" relationship. That is obvious, but the relationship is one of pure love. This dog has not only added greatly to our life as a family, but added *enormously* to Diana's. **Sometimes it's <u>not</u> OK to just say "No!"**

Like Duke and I, Bryan and Duchess will have a lifelong bond that will enhance his life forever.

Duchess never bit any of the children or their friends, shed very little and once even defended Diana from a stray dog. For sure, Diana was right when she said that she would end up being the one who would take care of Duchess, even though Bryan did more than a child's share of dog chores.

Holding on to your dreams as Bryan did, and believing they will come true is sometimes the difference between success in a quest and failure.

Compromise is the nature of all relationships. Sometimes when you totally give in like Diana did, you really end up getting more than you could have ever imagined.

Do I believe in signs? You bet I do.

Bryan & Duchess

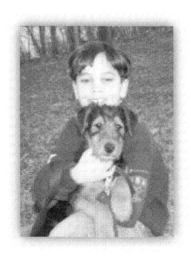

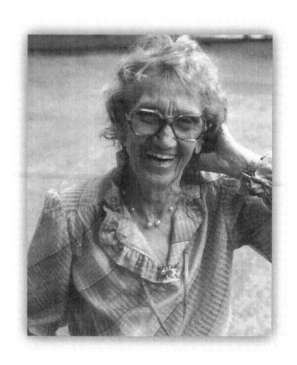

Mary at 90+

What Happens Now

In January 2010 a CT scan revealed three new areas of cancer growth. After several times of being informed of recurrence, our level of grief was quickly turned into proactive motivation. We rechecked with all our sources and doctors and at this point in time, there is no active treatment to be performed. The lesions are in areas that do not interfere with any bodily functions, and at this writing, we are weighing our options. The following life story demonstrates why we are confident of my survival.

Mary C., whose house neighbored my dental office, was over 100 years old when she passed away. I would often visit her over lunchtime long before cancer crossed my path. One day I asked her a question I'd been wondering about since we'd met: "Mary," I said, "You have lived a long and adventurous life. You have seven children, more than 20 grandchildren, almost 30 great-grandchildren and even a few great-great-grandchildren. What is your secret of living a long life?"

"God has a plan for everyone. He won't take you home until you accomplish what you are supposed to do down here," she said.

That sounded like some reasonable spiritual logic.

Then she leaned forward almost whispering in my ear while her eyes looked upward and said, "I'm not going to do it."

Then she smiled warmly, firm in her conviction with her intimacy with God, and believing that she was granted more time down here because she continued to be an active participant in life.

So the way I figure it, if that logic worked for Mary, I prey that it will work for me. There are so many things I have yet to accomplish.

As I said in the introduction, *you* are now part of my private militia. It is up to you to keep me down here spreading faith, encouragement and motivational stories. If you feel as though my stories will help someone who needs a boost, give them this book.

And please, keep me in your prayers. I know that may sound solicitous, but this is a battle for my life and I desire to stick around for a long, long time. Thank you.

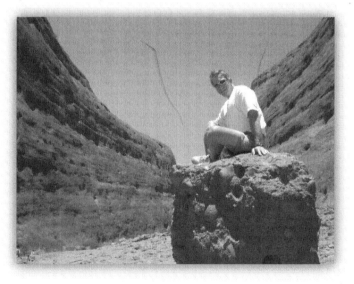

Me in Australia

Made in the USA
Charleston, SC
29 October 2010